THE CARNIVORE DIET FOR BEGINNERS

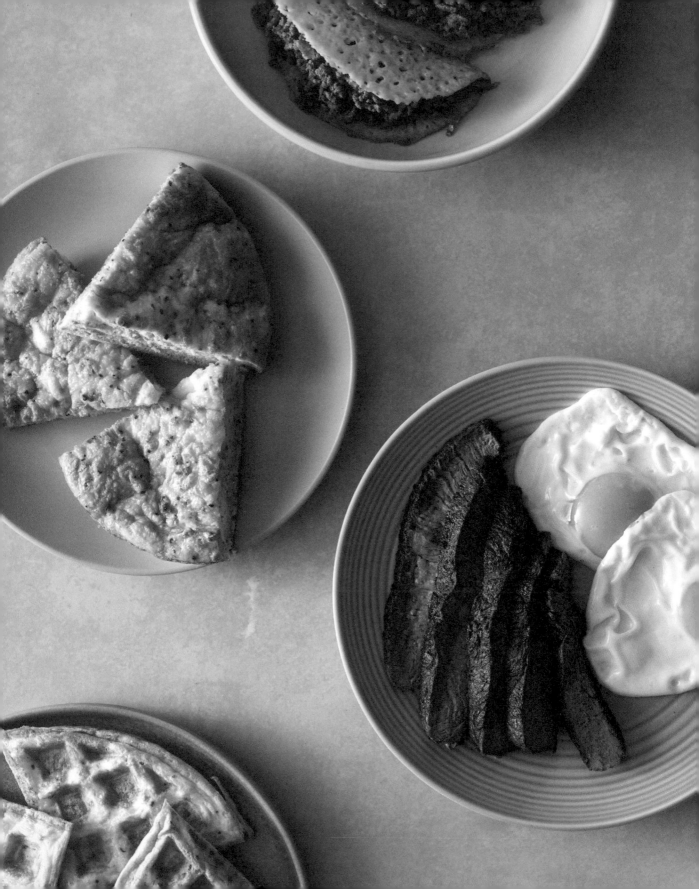

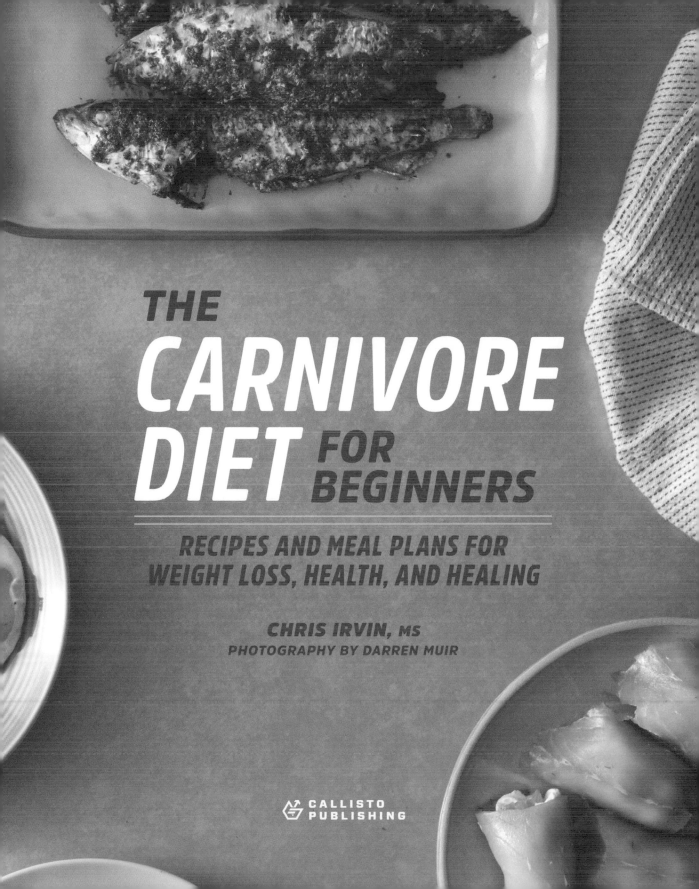

THE
CARNIVORE
DIET FOR BEGINNERS

RECIPES AND MEAL PLANS FOR WEIGHT LOSS, HEALTH, AND HEALING

CHRIS IRVIN, MS
PHOTOGRAPHY BY DARREN MUIR

CALLISTO
PUBLISHING

Copyright © 2021 by Callisto Publishing LLC
Cover and internal design © 2021 by Callisto Publishing LLC
Photography © 2021 Darren Muir; food styling by Yolanda Muir
Art Director: Patricia Fabricant
Art Producer: Meg Baggott
Editor: Justin Hartung
Production Editor: Emily Sheehan
Production Manager: Martin Worthington

Callisto Publishing and the colophon are registered trademarks of Callisto Publishing LLC

Published by Callisto Publishing LLC C/O Sourcebooks LLC
P.O. Box 4410, Naperville, Illinois 60567-4410
(630) 961-3900
callistopublishing.com

Printed and bound in China.
OGP 13

This book is dedicated to the many individuals suffering from autoimmune and digestive health issues. May you find health and healing in the carnivore diet.

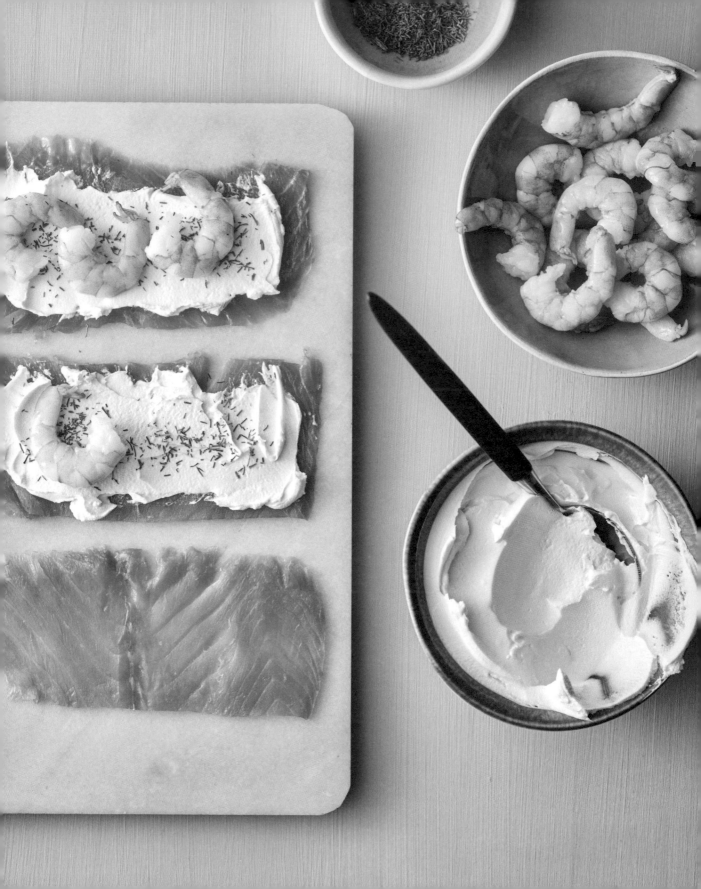

CONTENTS

INTRODUCTION ≡≡≡

I first became aware that the food I put in my body actually impacts my performance in life when I was a freshman in college. I was playing for my college's basketball team and happened to be taking my first nutrition class at the same time. That class opened my eyes to the fact that what I did in the kitchen (or, rather, the college cafeteria) could impact the way I performed on the court. This realization led me to focus on my diet throughout college—and forced me to learn from a lot of mistakes along the way.

After my undergraduate studies and taking some time off from school to train athletes, I decided to return to working toward my master's in nutrition science. This program pulled me deeper down the nutrition-science rabbit hole and introduced me to the ketogenic diet for the first time. After being blown away by the science of the keto diet and the results I was seeing while on it, I dove headfirst into studying the impact of low-carb and keto diets on athletic performance, human performance, and therapeutic intervention.

By the time I finished my master's degree, the keto diet had hit the mainstream. Now there were a ton of health professionals and social media influencers promoting the diet and new keto-labeled products coming to the market. Although there were definitely some cons to this boom with a spread of misinformation and industries trying to take advantage, there were also many pros due to the diet's ability to so profoundly affect our health.

During this time, I continued to study nutrition research, especially low-carb analysis, and create content to educate people about my findings. One day, I came across a diet I had never heard of or considered. I was listening to someone speak about the carnivore diet, which had helped both him and his daughter see profound improvements in their health.

At first, I was pretty skeptical. Surely, an all-meat diet couldn't be the optimal dietary approach for . . . well, anything. It seemed outrageous, but the more I heard people share their success stories with the diet and the more I dug into the research, the more I realized it wasn't as out there as I had originally thought.

Being a self-experimentation type of guy, I decided to give the diet a try. Coming from a low-carb diet, I didn't expect the carnivore diet to really provide me with much additional benefit, but I was wrong. Within a few days of eating like a carnivore, I started experiencing another level of mental clarity. I also noticed that my hunger levels were in check, allowing me to focus on work for longer periods of time, and my overall mood had improved. After continuing to follow the diet, I found that I not only started shedding body fat, but I also started putting on muscle. I even got my blood work done and was blown away to see that my cholesterol and triglyceride numbers weren't through the roof.

My experience, plus the countless hours spent reading literature available on the topic, has made me believe that a carnivore diet is a great option for numerous health goals, which is why I keep this diet technique in my tool kit to break out when I have a certain goal I am trying to achieve. In this book, I am going to teach you how to do the same. Whether you are looking to reset your gut, tackle autoimmune conditions, or lose weight, this book will lay out the science of—and, most importantly, the application for—a properly formulated carnivore diet.

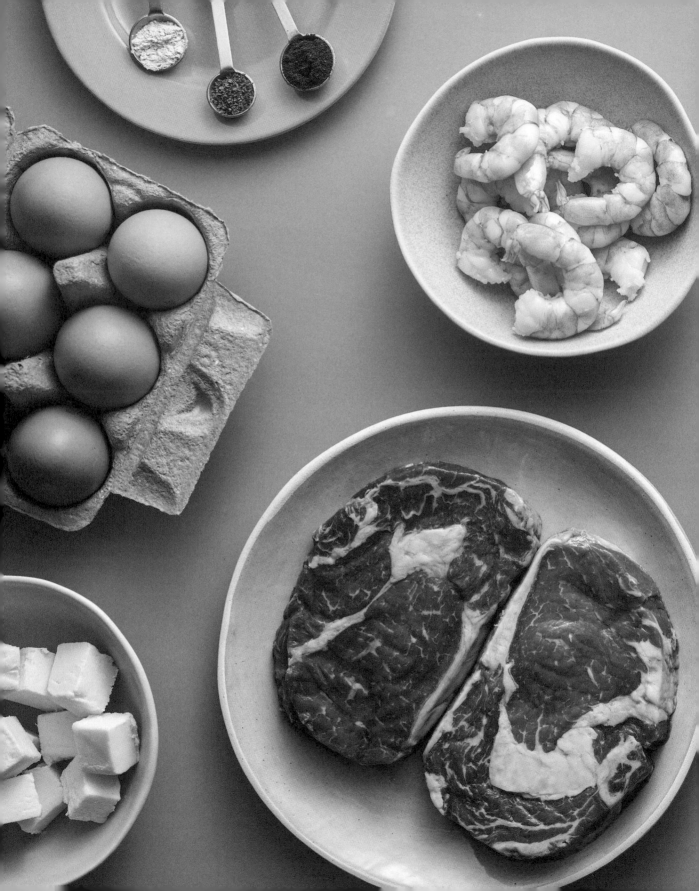

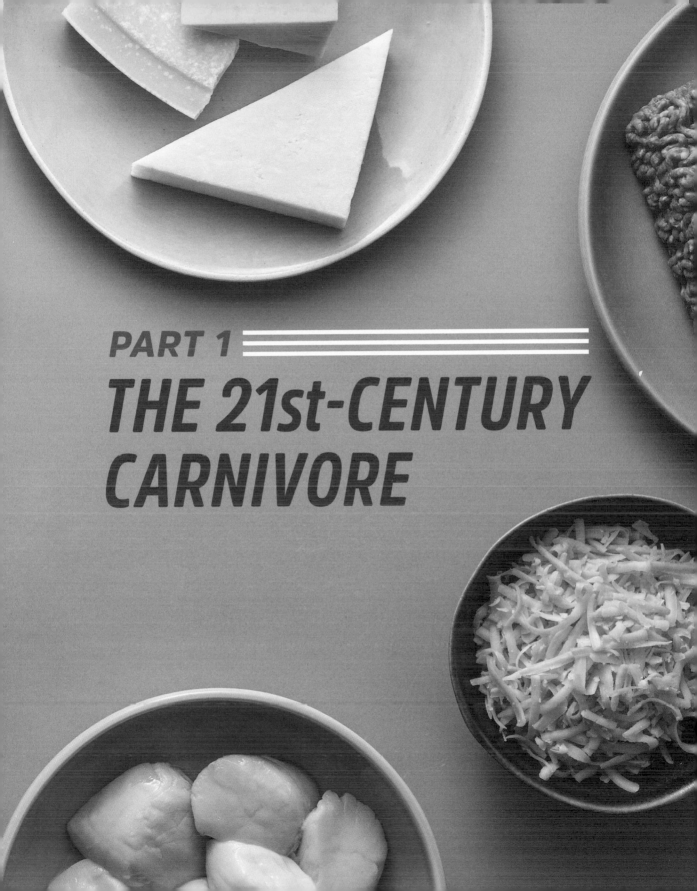

PART 1
THE 21st-CENTURY CARNIVORE

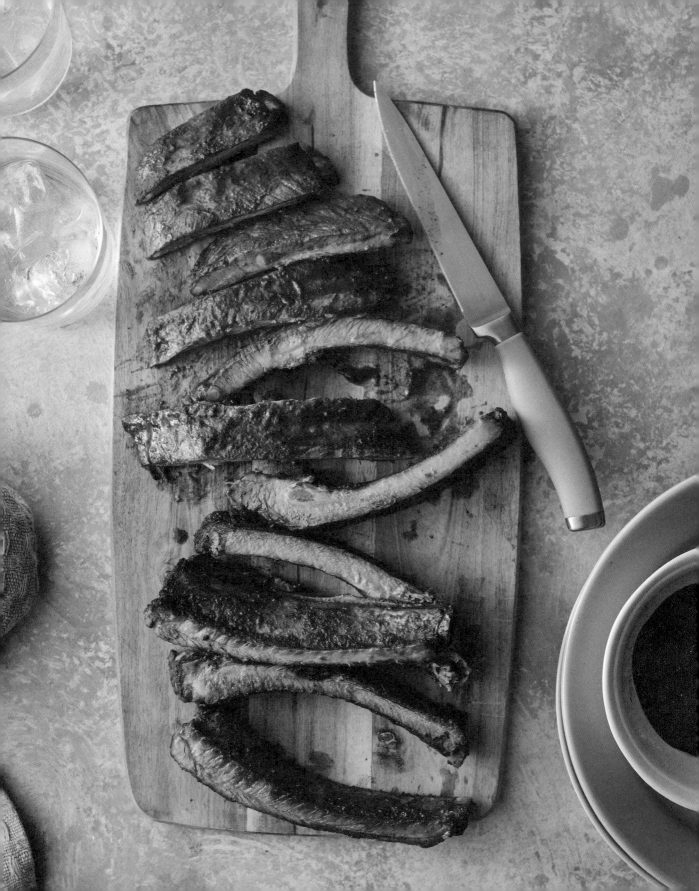

CHAPTER 1

UNDERSTANDING THE CARNIVORE DIET

A basic understanding of nutrition science will improve your chances of success on the carnivore diet. In this chapter, you'll learn the science supporting the diet along with its rich cultural history.

SLOW COOKER RIBS, PAGE 81

THE DEFINITION OF EATING CARNIVORE

You're probably thinking that defining *carnivore* can't be that hard. You simply eat meat, right? Although that is a key component to the diet, there is a little more to it than meets the eye. A carnivore diet is not just a meat-based diet. It is an animal-based diet. Depending on your goals and specific reasons for following carnivore, other foods produced by animals can be incorporated into your diet to help contribute to your nutrient intake and add some extra flavor. Here are the different food categories that make up a carnivore diet.

MEAT

Meat should make up 90 percent or more of your carnivore diet and includes beef, pork, chicken, fish, and even game such as bison, venison, and elk. However, when it comes to choosing meat on a carnivore diet, red meat should be your go-to. It's incredibly nutrient dense because it comes from ruminant animals (animals with multiple stomachs), which have the ability to break down plants and harness their nutrients in their meat, meaning you can better absorb them than if you ate the plants yourself. It's in your best interest to opt for beef, bison, or elk whenever you can.

It's impossible to discuss meat without giving a shout-out to organ meat. Liver, heart, and kidney are packed with nutrients—they're essentially a carnivore dieter's multivitamin. Organ meats do not have to be a staple of your diet, but an optimized carnivore diet will include organs at least once a week.

ANIMAL FAT (FOR COOKING)

Arguably the biggest issue with the standard American diet is the choice of cooking oils. Nearly every restaurant you go to is cooking your food in inflammatory vegetable oils such as canola, corn, soybean, or safflower oil. These oils are loaded with omega-6 fats that become damaged during production. When foods are fried in these oils, you're introduced to a heavy toxic load that can drive up inflammation—and even contribute to insulin resistance.

On a carnivore diet, you avoid these oils and instead opt for animal fats such as butter, tallow, and lard. These fats contain beneficial nutrients and have a higher smoke point, which prevents them from oxidizing and becoming damaged when you cook with them. Animal fat also contributes an additional flavor boost to your carnivore recipes. The recipes in this book call for salted butter, but you can swap it for tallow or lard if you prefer.

SALT AND SPICES

While salt and spices are not animal-based, they *do* help add flavor to this way of eating. Turmeric, basil, garlic, sage, and thyme can expand your palate on carnivore to keep things interesting. However, if you are following a carnivore diet to treat autoimmune or gut health issues, you may want to opt for no spices to avoid any potential flare-ups these ingredients could cause to an already damaged gut.

Salt is a key addition to carnivore because sodium is an electrolyte that becomes depleted when you eat a low-carb diet. Sodium is a key regulator of hundreds of functions in the body, so you can't perform optimally when you're depleted of it. If you're into the ancestral way of eating, you may be wondering if your predecessors had to salt their meat. Actually, some sources suggest they drank the blood of animals, which is rich in electrolytes like sodium. Unless you are going the blood-drinking route, be sure to season your food with some salt to help replenish this crucial electrolyte as well as enhance the flavor.

DAIRY AND EGGS

Dairy and eggs contain a nearly 1:1 fat-to-protein ratio, making them useful tools for increasing your fat intake on carnivore. Eggs are incredibly nutrient dense and are a complete source of protein. They are one of the few foods I would actually classify as a superfood. (Organ meat is another.) Dairy can add some benefits as well, but it is much harder to source. Most store-bought dairy has been highly processed and is thus devoid of the majority of its beneficial nutrients. Choose raw (unpasteurized) dairy when you can, which you can usually find at your local farmers' market.

Both dairy and eggs can trigger gut flare-ups in some individuals, which is why you won't find either in the first week of the carnivore elimination meal plan coming up in the next chapter. Many people find that if these foods have given them problems in the past, a few weeks of carnivore is enough to reset their gut and allow for these foods to be reincorporated into their diet.

BONE BROTH AND OTHER BEVERAGES

Bone broth is another great resource on the carnivore diet. Bone broth is rich in the amino acid glycine, which is difficult to get in your diet otherwise. Glycine plays many roles in the body but can most notably promote stronger hair, skin, and nails and even contribute to gut restoration and better digestive health. Bone broth is also a rich source of sodium, further contributing to electrolyte replenishment on the diet.

There are not many other beverages that fall into the carnivore category besides water. Drinks such as coffee and alcohol may be tolerated in low doses on carnivore, but note these are not of animal origin and should be avoided during the elimination phase of the diet.

THE ORIGINAL CARNIVORES

Although many consider carnivore a more recent diet, its roots go much deeper. We first saw carnivore pop up as a diet trend in 1856 when German writer Bernard Moncriff published the book *The Philosophy of the Stomach; or, An Exclusively Animal Diet: The Most Wholesome and Fit for Man*, arguing that an animal-based diet was superior to both a mixed diet and a plant-based diet for health.

Despite Moncriff being one of the first to address carnivore as a diet, animal-based eating has a rich ancestral history. There is much evidence that some Neanderthals were primarily meat-eaters. And many societies throughout history have consumed organs, with nutrient-rich liver being the first food they would reach for after long periods of not eating.

This brief look at ancestral dieting is not meant to convince you that all of your ancestors ate only meat. Historically speaking, diet was much more dependent on location—you ate what was available to you. Therefore, there are also ancestral groups that were plant-based and mixed dieters. But carnivore is a diet that humans have thrived off of in the past, and so can you.

CARNIVORE AS AN ELIMINATION DIET

One of the best uses of carnivore is as an elimination diet, which removes all potential toxins and triggers that could be impairing your digestive health. There are many other elimination diets out there, but what makes carnivore so special is that it removes *all* potential triggers to allow your gut to rest and provides an array of nutrients that your digestive system can use to repair and strengthen itself along the way.

The benefits of carnivore don't stop at digestive health. Using carnivore as an elimination diet can positively impact your health in numerous other ways. Here are the most notable.

WEIGHT LOSS

Weight loss can be a primary goal of carnivore or a great complementary benefit. Carnivore often leads to weight loss similar to the way the ketogenic diet does: through carbohydrate restriction. Carb restriction lowers your blood sugar and insulin levels, which is more conducive to fat burning. When you follow a low-carb diet such as carnivore, your body transitions from using carbs to using stored body fat for fuel.

Carnivore can also improve metabolism and digestion, which further support weight loss. The lack of hunger (also known as satiety) that typically accompanies this way of eating is another key player in weight loss as it prevents you from overeating.

AUTOIMMUNE HEALING

The carnivore diet as a way to manage autoimmune disease is likely the most promising therapeutic application of this diet. Whether source or symptom, impaired digestive health is a key contributor to autoimmune disease. When you eliminate foods that cause your gut to flare up, you can improve symptoms of many autoimmune conditions. Plants are a huge source of anti-nutrients such as phytates, oxalates, and saponins, which can wreak havoc on an already-damaged gut. On a carnivore diet, you are giving your digestive system a break from these potentially harmful compounds so your gut can restore itself.

SIMPLE, MORE ACCESSIBLE DIETING

The first time I tried carnivore, I saw a tremendous amount of success. I lost weight, I was more energetic, and I felt a lot stronger in the gym. One of the benefits I enjoyed the most was the boost in productivity I experienced. I noticed that when I was on carnivore, I never really thought about food. I would have to remind myself to eat and did very little snacking between meals. Meal prep on carnivore was also much easier, and it gave me a lot more time to focus on research and writing.

The lack of hunger you experience on carnivore is a result of many mechanisms, including a less palatable diet. Don't get me wrong, steak is delicious. But it doesn't have the same impact on your brain's reward centers as super sweet and savory foods do. This works to your advantage because you start to actually register fullness while you are eating, and your hunger signals begin to operate the way they should.

IMPORTANT NOTE

Before digging in too far, it is crucial to point out that more research is needed on the long-term effects of a carnivore diet. Existing research provides the effects of eating meat and the health of ancestors who ate meat, but no recent randomized controlled clinical trials have been done on the carnivore diet. Although there is also no sufficient scientific evidence that carnivore is dangerous, be aware of how your body responds as you begin the diet so you can assess if it's right for you.

NUTRITION ON THE CARNIVORE DIET

The carnivore diet falls into the larger diet classification of low carb. When you are eating primarily meat, your carbohydrate intake is so low that it is likely you will induce at least a minor state of ketosis, leading many to refer to this diet as carnivore keto.

When you reduce carb intake, you give overused parts of your metabolic machinery a rest, allowing blood sugar to normalize, insulin levels to drop, and your body to restore its ability to respond to insulin. (A hormone produced by the pancreas in response to carbohydrate consumption, insulin's role is to help sugar get from the blood into the cell to be used for energy. When this process is overstimulated, insulin resistance occurs, and cells lose their ability to respond to insulin.) This also results in ketosis, or the production of ketone bodies, which are little molecules that provide you with energy and downstream benefits such as repaired metabolism, better brain health and function, and even lower inflammation.

WHO SHOULD NOT FOLLOW THE CARNIVORE DIET?

The carnivore diet sounds really great, doesn't it? But you may be wondering if this diet is for everyone. To really answer this question, it needs to be broken down into two separate questions:

Is the carnivore diet safe for everyone?

The diet is safe for almost everyone. Those with conditions requiring lower protein intake or those who are prone to a poor response when making a major diet shift (such as pregnant people) should consult a knowledgeable physician before trying the carnivore diet.

Is the carnivore diet the best option for everyone?

No. The carnivore diet is not the best option for everyone. If you already have strong metabolic and digestive health and are consuming a nutrient- and protein-rich diet, the added benefit of a carnivore diet may be minor at best. If you have a history of eating disorders or a poor relationship with food, this diet may not be the right fit for you due to its restrictive nature.

Remember that nutrition should always be personalized based on what is best for the individual. Carnivore is a great nutrition tool that can be used to help you achieve specific goals in certain situations, but it is not an end-all-be-all diet that you must follow forever.

One of the biggest differences between carnivore and keto is the amount of protein consumed. Traditionally speaking, keto has placed an emphasis on keeping protein intake lower, around 25 percent of total calories. On a carnivore diet, your protein intake will be much higher. Protein is used for building structural components of your body and plays a role in nearly every bodily function. Long story short, you'll be putting this extra protein to good use.

NUTRIENT DENSITY AND BIOAVAILABILITY

Nutrient density accounts for many of the benefits experienced on a carnivore diet. Meat is packed with B vitamins, vitamin D_3, DHA, heme iron, cholesterol, and unique amino acids like taurine, leucine, and creatine—all critical and beneficial nutrients that are not found in plants. Organ meats are nature's multivitamin, providing the aforementioned nutrients, plus vitamin A, choline, copper, folate, and many more. Meat and eggs are also loaded with beneficial fats and are complete protein sources, meaning they contain all of the essential amino acids you require, including those critical for muscle growth.

What makes the nutrient density of meat so impactful is its *bioavailability*. Bioavailability is a term used to describe the amount your body can absorb of a nutrient or compound. It does not matter if a food is packed with nutrients if they are not bioavailable. You simply can't use nutrients you can't absorb. Ruminant animals (cows, bison, and elk) have digestive systems that make plants very bioavailable to them. They can break down these plants and convert them into nutrients that are stored in their tissues. The form these nutrients take when harnessed in animal tissue allows them to be more bioavailable to humans because we have different digestive systems. In other words, you better absorb the nutrients found in animal protein than the ones found in plants. Nutrient density plus superior bioavailability equals optimal human function.

DAILY CALORIE INTAKE

Calories play a role in any diet, and carnivore is no exception. However, carnivore does not focus on caloric intake the way other diets do.

You tend to have less hunger and fewer cravings when you are eating only meat because of the higher protein and fat intake, being in ketosis, and the lack of overly sweet or savory flavors that can trigger a hunger response. This typically prevents people from overeating on carnivore without having to count calories. However, this lack of hunger does present the risk of undereating. My recommendation is to shoot for one gram of protein per pound of body weight per day, and if you need to eat more calories, make sure that protein is coming from fattier cuts of meat (or vice versa if you need to eat fewer calories). It may be beneficial to track your calories at first to understand what a day of eating should look like for you.

THE ROLE OF FIBER

A common concern with a carnivore diet is fiber. How can a diet that has virtually no fiber in it be healthy? There is actually no scientific evidence that says you need fiber. In fact, even the research suggesting the benefits of fiber is flawed. Typically, these studies will take someone on a standard American diet who regularly consumes processed food and have them replace part of their diet with high-fiber foods. When this elicits some kind of measurable benefit, the study reports that fiber caused that benefit. But doesn't it make sense that trading a fast-food burger and fries for broccoli is going to induce some health benefits? Does this mean it was all about the fiber?

Interestingly, there is some research suggesting that lowering fiber intake can actually improve digestive symptoms for those suffering from constipation. While this may seem counterintuitive, too much fiber can cause digestive distress in the same way it was thought too little fiber could. This is not to say that fiber is unhealthy or that it has no benefits. But if you are following this diet with goals of improving your digestive health or tackling autoimmune symptoms, the break from fiber may be exactly what your body needs.

≡ WILL I NEED SUPPLEMENTS?

Supplements should never be required for a diet to be successful. Instead, supplements should be used to complement a diet or to fill a gap that is present because of your specific approach to the diet. The need for supplements on carnivore is very low considering the nutrient density and bioavailability mentioned earlier. However, there are some supplements that can be helpful.

ELECTROLYTES: Essential to every function in the human body, electrolytes are typically deficient in most diets because you don't drink blood. An electrolyte supplement such as Perfect Keto or LMNT may be helpful, but note that these supplements are not totally carnivore (see Resources, page 108).

COLLAGEN: Collagen is a protein that contains the unique amino acids glycine, proline, and hydroxyproline, which are beneficial to your connective tissues and are hard to get in your diet unless you are eating animal connective tissue.

PROTEIN POWDER: Animal-based protein powders such as beef, whey, and egg protein are an easy way to help you reach your protein goals. Be sure to check the labels to avoid additives.

ORGAN CAPSULES: Not everyone loves organ meat, which is why organ meat capsules may be a great alternative. However, I would not consider this to be superior to consuming the whole-food form of organ meat.

COMMON ISSUES DURING THE ELIMINATION DIET

Although the carnivore diet is a safe diet, some symptoms often accompany its induction. The most notable are fatigue and muscle cramps. If you are familiar with keto, these symptoms are very similar to the "keto flu." Just like keto, the low-carb nature of a carnivore diet lowers your insulin levels, which can increase water and electrolyte excretion, leading to dehydration. A great way to combat this is by drinking plenty of water, salting your foods, and maybe even using an electrolyte supplement.

It is also common to experience changes in your bowel movements at the start of carnivore. This big change in diet and the removal of fiber can lead to short-term loose stools. For most people, this subsides after a few days to a couple of weeks as your body adjusts and becomes more accustomed to this new way of eating.

Another common cause of issues on carnivore is the overconsumption of *processed* red meats such as bacon, packaged sausage, and deli meat. Like any diet, the quality of your carnivore is important. Processed red meats are much lower quality, contain harmful fillers and preservatives, and have fewer beneficial nutrients. This can contribute to digestive distress and prevent you from seeing all of the health benefits this diet has to offer.

In general, most of the symptoms experienced at the beginning of carnivore will subside quickly, especially if you are focusing on consuming high-quality animal protein, staying hydrated, and replenishing your electrolytes.

HOLISTIC HEALTH

Although nutrition is one of the biggest levers we can pull to improve our health, there are numerous other factors of health that should not be overlooked. These lifestyle factors include exercise, sleep, and stress management. If you are eating a healthy diet but ignoring these factors, you are leaving health improvements on the table.

How you move your body, your sleep habits, and your exposure to stress also play a key role in how your body responds to your diet and your ability to adhere to that diet. For instance, having high levels of cortisol from stress can make it harder to burn fat, lack of exercise can lead to poor mood (making it harder to have the discipline to stick to a diet), and poor sleep can worsen the function of your digestive system and even make you more likely to make poor food choices throughout the day.

Strive to look at your health more holistically. Understand that the best health plan is the one that couples strong nutrition principles with exercise, quality sleep, and proper stress management techniques. Mastering each of these components of health will require intention and discipline, but committing to subtle improvements in these areas will make a big difference in your diet and health as a whole.

≡ SOURCING THE HIGHEST-QUALITY MEAT

A lot of research has been dedicated to debunking the health myths around red meat and fat, but there hasn't been much focus on debunking the myths around the environmental impacts of meat. Meat has been demonized for destroying our environment, but if you look at the science, these claims have been drastically overblown. However, some animal agriculture practices are better for the environment than others.

Animals produced under regenerative agriculture models not only provide a higher-quality meat but also help improve the health of the environment along the way. When you source any food, including meat, you are voting with your dollars. What do you want to be supporting with your hard-earned money? Big corporations that don't have your health in mind? Or local farmers doing what they can for the health of their local community, environment, and economy?

To support better environmental practices:

▶ Source from local farmers and farmers' markets
▶ Look for grass-fed meats at your grocery store
▶ Join a meat delivery service such as ButcherBox
▶ Order Force of Nature Meats or White Oak Pastures online

See Resources (page 108) for more about these products.

To learn more about the environmental impact of meat, check out the book *Sacred Cow* by Robb Wolf and Diana Rodgers.

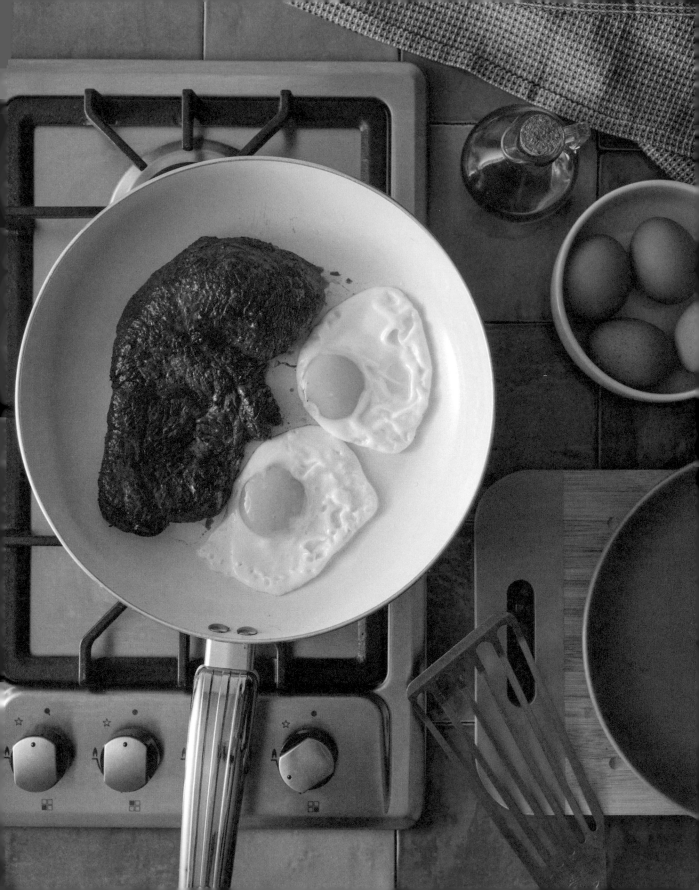

CHAPTER 2

THE 4-WEEK CARNIVORE ELIMINATION PLAN

An elimination diet removes all foods with toxins and gut-damaging compounds to allow your digestive system to rest and recover. The added benefit of a carnivore elimination diet is that red meat contains nutrients that strengthen your digestive system.

STEAK AND EGGS, PAGE **28**

Dairy, eggs, and plant-based seasonings can trigger digestive responses in some individuals, especially those with impaired gut health. For this reason, the four-week elimination plan outlined in this chapter will start with just meat and slowly add back eggs, dairy, and seasonings as tolerated by your body.

Here is an overview of what the four-week elimination plan will look like:

WEEK 1: Meat and Salt

WEEK 2: Meat and Eggs

WEEK 3: Meat, Eggs, Dairy

WEEK 4: Meat, Eggs, Dairy, Seasonings

If you are giving carnivore a try to reduce autoimmune symptoms, you may need to stay on a stricter regimen for longer. This is because you may be more prone to reactions to eggs, dairy, and especially seasonings. Always assess your reactions to foods and don't be afraid to consult with a physician who properly understands this diet, such as an alternative medicine doctor or a doctor who specializes in a low-carb lifestyle (see Resources, page 108).

Note that this meal plan was constructed to serve one person and uses leftovers with that in mind. If you are cooking for more than just yourself, consider the serving sizes of each recipe when meal prepping for the week. The beginning of this elimination diet will be extremely simple; to keep things interesting, opt for different cuts of meat from various animals, such as rib eye, New York strip, pork chops, ground pork, and so on. As the weeks go by, you will be able to add more and more variety to help keep your carnivore diet new and delicious!

WEEK 1	BREAKFAST	LUNCH	DINNER
SUNDAY	Ground Breakfast Boar (page 26)	Bacon-Wrapped Pork Medallions (page 88)	Chicken Skewers (page 71)
MONDAY	Breakfast Steak (page 27)	Bacon-Wrapped Pork Medallions *leftovers*	Whole Baked Chicken (page 67)
TUESDAY	Ground Breakfast Boar (page 26)	Pan-Seared Bone-In Rib Eye (page 90)	Chicken Skewers *leftovers*
WEDNESDAY	Ground Breakfast Boar (page 26)	Whole Baked Chicken *leftovers*	Bacon-Wrapped Pork Medallions *leftovers*
THURSDAY	Breakfast Steak (page 27)	Beef Heart and Liver Meatballs (page 100)	Bacon Scallop Skewers (page 53)
FRIDAY	Ground Breakfast Boar (page 26)	Whole Baked Chicken *leftovers*	Beef Heart and Liver Meatballs *leftovers*
SATURDAY	Breakfast Steak (page 27)	Bacon-Wrapped Chicken Tenders (page 69)	Bacon Scallop Skewers (page 53)

SNACKS: Leftovers of Whole Baked Chicken, Pan-Seared Bone-In Rib Eye, and Beef Heart and Liver Meatballs

SHOPPING LIST

MEAT

- Bacon, 3 (16-ounce) packages
- Beef, ground (8 ounces)
- Beef, ground heart (4 ounces)
- Beef, ground liver (4 ounces)
- Boar, ground (2 pounds)
- Chicken, boneless, skinless breasts (1 pound)
- Chicken, tenders (1 pound)
- Chicken, whole (6 pounds)
- Pork, 1 (1-pound) tenderloin
- Rib-eye, 2 (8-ounce) bone-in steaks, 1 inch thick
- Strip, 3 (8-ounce) steaks

SEAFOOD

- 8 scallops

PANTRY

- Sea salt

WEEK 2	BREAKFAST	LUNCH	DINNER
SUNDAY	Ground Breakfast Boar (page 26)	Pan-Seared Bone-In Rib Eye (page 90)	Bacon-Wrapped Shrimp (page 59)
MONDAY	Egg and Bacon Rollup (page 34)	Sunny-Side-Up Burger (page 89)	Pan-Seared Bone-In Rib Eye *leftovers*
TUESDAY	Sausage Egg in a Basket (page 35)	Bacon-Wrapped Shrimp *leftovers*	Baked Chicken Drumsticks (page 75)
WEDNESDAY	Egg and Bacon Rollup (page 34)	Baked Chicken Drumsticks *leftovers*	Beef Heart Skewers (page 99)
THURSDAY	Breakfast Steak (page 27)	Chicken Skewers (page 71)	Beef Heart Skewers *leftovers*
FRIDAY	Ground Breakfast Boar (page 26)	Chicken Skewers *leftovers*	Bacon-Wrapped Pork Medallions (page 88)
SATURDAY	Sausage Egg in a Basket (page 35)	Bacon-Wrapped Pork Medallions *leftovers*	Pan-Seared Bone-In Rib Eye (page 90)

SNACKS: Leftovers of Bacon-Wrapped Shrimp, Bacon-Wrapped Pork Medallions, and Pan-Seared Bone-In Rib Eye or hard-boiled eggs

SHOPPING LIST

MEAT

- Bacon, 3 (16-ounce) packages
- Beef, ground (5 ounces)
- Beef, 1 heart
- Boar, ground (1 pound)
- Chicken, boneless, skinless breasts (1 pound)
- Chicken, drumsticks (1 pound)
- Pork, ground, breakfast sausage (8 ounces)
- Pork, 1 (1-pound) tenderloin
- Rib-eye, 4 (8-ounce) bone-in steaks, 1 inch thick
- Strip, 1 (8-ounce) steak

SEAFOOD

- Shrimp, peeled, deveined (1 pound)

EGGS AND DAIRY

- Eggs (1 dozen)

PANTRY

- Sea salt

WEEK 3	BREAKFAST	LUNCH	DINNER
SUNDAY	Chaffle Breakfast Sandwich (page 32)	Bacon Buck Burger (page 97)	Parmesan-Crusted Cod (page 60)
MONDAY	Chaffle Breakfast Sandwich leftovers	Bacon Buck Burger leftovers	"Breaded" Pork Chops (page 91)
TUESDAY	Bacon and Feta Omelet (page 33)	"Breaded" Pork Chops leftovers	Beef Liver Pâté (page 102)
WEDNESDAY	Sausage Egg Cups (page 30)	Brown Butter Mahi-Mahi (page 54)	Bacon Buck Burger leftovers
THURSDAY	Egg and Bacon Rollup (page 34)	"Breaded" Pork Chops leftovers	Cheesy Chicken Quesadilla (page 72)
FRIDAY	Sausage Egg Cups leftovers	Tuna Chaffle Melt (page 58)	Beef Liver Pâté leftovers
SATURDAY	Sausage Egg Cups leftovers	Sautéed Beef Kidney (page 103)	Tuna Chaffle Melt leftovers

SNACKS: Leftovers of Bacon Buck Burgers, "Breaded" Pork Chops, Beef Liver Pâté, and Sausage Egg Cups. You can also snack on Fried Deviled Eggs (page 42), Bacon-Wrapped Mozzarella (page 40), or Cream Cheese Sausage Balls (page 47).

SHOPPING LIST

MEAT

- Bacon, 2 (16-ounce) packages
- Beef, 1 kidney
- Beef, liver (½ pound)
- Chicken, 1 (6-ounce) boneless, skinless breast

- Pork, 4 (6-ounce) boneless chops
- Pork, ground, breakfast sausage (1 pound)
- Venison, ground (1 pound)

SEAFOOD

- Cod, 1 (8-ounce) fillet

- Mahi-mahi, 1 (6-ounce) fillet

EGGS AND DAIRY

- Butter, salted (1 pound)
- Cheddar, cheese, shredded, 1 (16-ounce) bag

- Cheddar, cheese, slices, 1 (8-ounce) package
- Cream, heavy, whipping (1 pint)

CONTINUED >>

- Eggs (3 dozen)
- Feta, cheese, crumbles,
  1 (6-ounce) container
- Mozzarella, cheese, shredded,
  1 (16-ounce) bag

- Mozzarella, cheese, slices,
  1 (8-ounce) package
- Parmesan, cheese, grated,
  1 (8-ounce) container
- Parmesan, cheese, shredded,
  1 (8-ounce) container

PANTRY

- Pork rinds
- Sea salt

- Tuna, 1 (5-ounce) can

WEEK 4	BREAKFAST	LUNCH	DINNER
SUNDAY	Chaffle Breakfast Sandwich (page 32)	Creamy Garlic Shrimp (page 61)	Pulled Pork (page 80)
MONDAY	Chaffle Breakfast Sandwich *leftovers*	Bacon Buck Burger (page 97)	Creamy Garlic Shrimp *leftovers*
TUESDAY	Sausage and Goat Cheese Frittata (page 31)	Pulled Pork *leftovers*	Baked Cod (page 52)
WEDNESDAY	Steak and Eggs (page 28)	Cheesy Tacos (page 86)	Creamy Garlic Shrimp *leftovers*
THURSDAY	Sausage and Goat Cheese Frittata *leftovers*	Garlic Butter Steak Bites (page 79)	Pulled Pork *leftovers*
FRIDAY	Sausage and Goat Cheese Frittata *leftovers*	Egg Salad (page 41)	Cheesy Tacos *leftovers*
SATURDAY	Egg and Bacon Rollup (page 34)	Brown Butter Mahi-Mahi (page 54)	Chicken Salad Cannoli (page 68)

SNACKS: Leftovers of Bacon Buck Burgers and Chicken Salad Cannoli. You can also snack on Beef Jerky (page 38), Cheesy "Breadsticks" (page 44), or Fried Deviled Eggs (page 42).

SHOPPING LIST

MEAT

- Bacon, 2 (16-ounce) packages
- Beef, ground (½ pound)
- Chicken, boneless, skinless breasts (1 pound)
- Pork, ground, breakfast sausage (16 ounces)
- Pork, 1 (1-pound) loin
- Rib-eye, 1 (6-ounce) steak
- Rib-eye, 1 (8-ounce) steak
- Venison, ground (1 pound)

SEAFOOD

- Cod, 1 (4-ounce) fillet
- Mahi-mahi, 1 (6-ounce) fillet
- Shrimp, peeled, deveined, (1 pound)

EGGS AND DAIRY

- Butter, salted (1 pound)
- Cheddar, cheese, shredded, 1 (16-ounce) bag
- Cheddar, cheese, slices, 1 (8-ounce) package
- Cream cheese, 1 (8-ounce) carton
- Cream, heavy, whipping (1 pint)
- Eggs (2 dozen)
- Goat, cheese, crumbles, 1 (4-ounce) log
- Mozzarella, cheese, shredded, 1 (16-ounce) bag
- Parmesan, cheese, grated, 1 (8-ounce) container
- Sour cream, 1 (8-ounce) container

PANTRY

- Black pepper, freshly ground
- Chili, powder
- Cumin, powder
- Garlic, powder
- Onion, powder
- Oregano, dried
- Paprika, ground
- Parsley, dried
- Sea salt

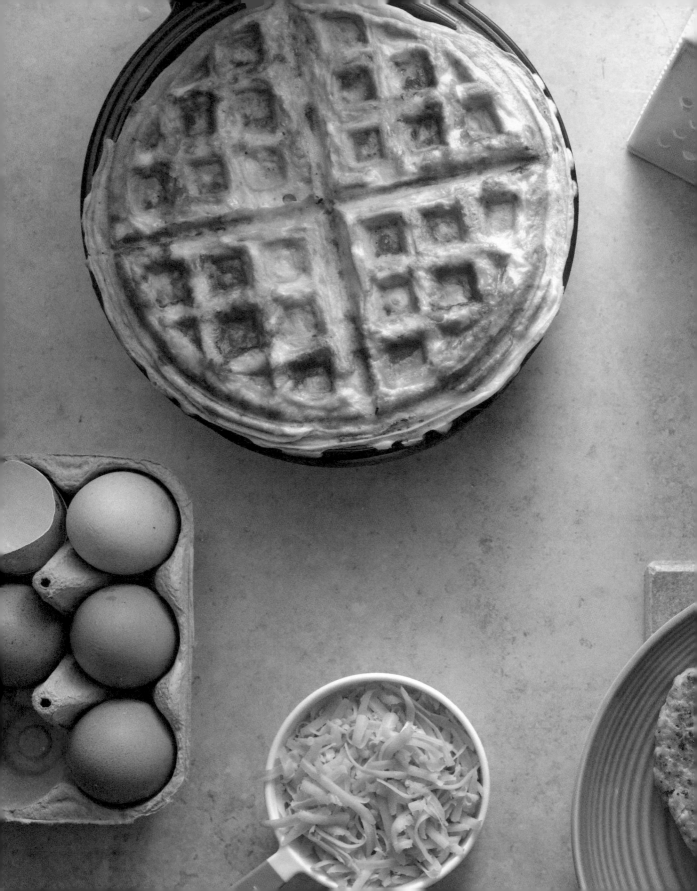

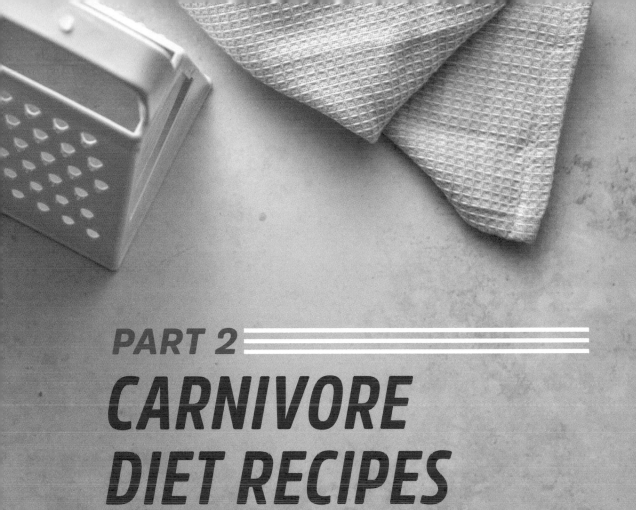

PART 2

CARNIVORE DIET RECIPES

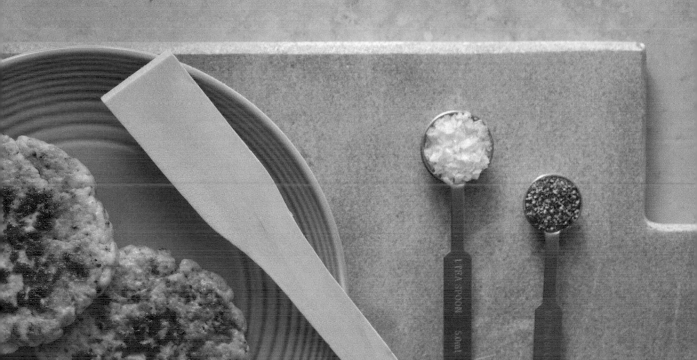

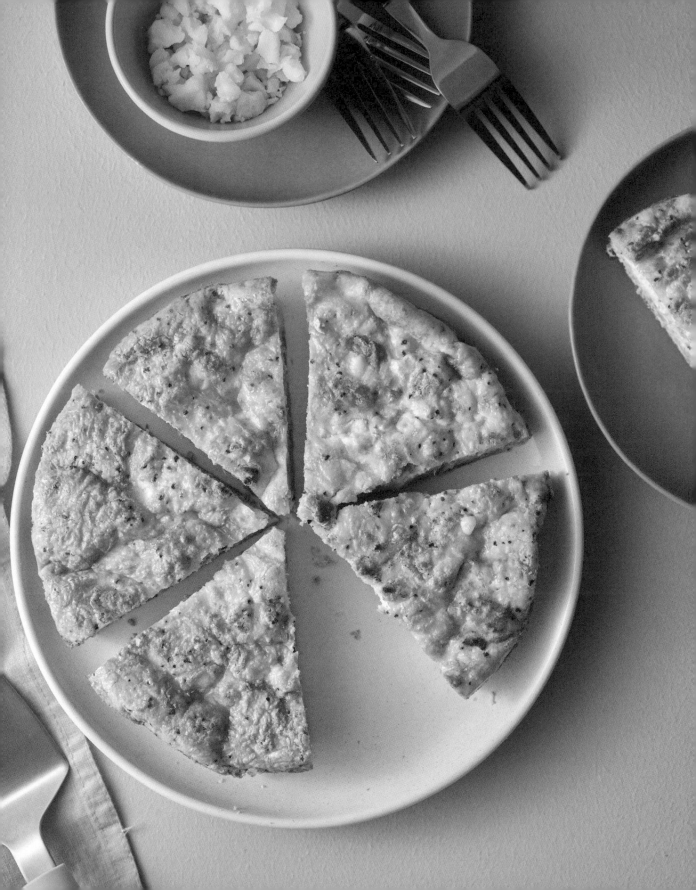

CHAPTER 3

BREAKFAST

GROUND BREAKFAST BOAR

SERVES 1 / COOK TIME: 10 minutes

DAIRY-FREE, EGG-FREE

Ground boar is incredibly flavorful, making it a great breakfast option during those meat-only stages of carnivore. I source mine at Force of Nature Meats (see Resources, page 108). Compared to commercial pork, wild boar is much leaner and has more protein. It's a great lower-calorie breakfast option for light morning eaters.

8 ounces ground boar

1 Set a small sauté pan over medium-high heat. Once hot, cook the ground boar, stirring to break up the meat, until browned, 6 to 8 minutes.

2 Serve immediately or store in an airtight container in the refrigerator for up to 3 days.

> **TIP:** The boar is fatty enough that you shouldn't need to grease the pan with butter, but if you're worried about sticking, use a nonstick sauté pan.

PER SERVING: Calories: 280; Fat: 8g; Carbohydrates: 0g; Protein: 48g; Sodium: 360mg; Iron: 4mg

BREAKFAST STEAK

SERVES 1 / COOK TIME: 10 minutes

EGG-FREE

Who doesn't love steak for breakfast? Another go-to for those only eating meat, steak is rich in protein and, depending on the cut you choose, high in fat—a great combo if you're needing looking for a morning energy boost that will last until lunch. Looking for a fattier breakfast? Swap the strip steak for rib eye.

1 tablespoon salted butter

1 (8-ounce) strip steak

1 In a small sauté pan, melt the butter over medium-high heat.

2 Add the steak and sear on both sides, 3 to 4 minutes per side, depending on your desired doneness.

3 Serve immediately or store in an airtight container in the refrigerator for up to 3 days.

TIP: If you're enjoying this steak during week 1 or 2 of the meal plan, omit the butter and use a nonstick pan.

PER SERVING: Calories: 530; Fat: 36g; Carbohydrates: 0g; Protein: 47g; Sodium: 212mg; Iron: 3mg

STEAK AND EGGS

SERVES 1 / COOK TIME: 10 minutes

Steak by itself is a great option for better absorption of protein and nutri-ents. Throw in a few eggs and you have a combo that provides you with ample protein, quality fat, nutrients, and compounds that support optimal brain function.

2 tablespoons salted butter, divided

1 (6-ounce) rib-eye steak

1 teaspoon sea salt, divided

½ teaspoon freshly ground black pepper, divided

1 teaspoon onion powder, divided

3 eggs, beaten

1 In a small sauté pan, melt 1 tablespoon of butter over medium-high heat.

2 Add the steak and season one side with ½ teaspoon of salt, ¼ teaspoon of pepper, and ½ teaspoon of onion powder. Cook until the steak has a nice sear on it, 3 to 4 minutes. Flip and season the other side with the remaining ½ teaspoon of salt, ¼ teaspoon of pepper, and ½ teaspoon of onion powder.

3 Immediately add the remaining 1 tablespoon of butter and eggs into the pan around the steak. Cook for 3 to 4 minutes, stirring the eggs to scramble them, until the steak reaches your desired doneness and the eggs are no longer runny.

4 Serve or store in an airtight container in the refrigerator for up to 3 days.

TIP: Try sunny-side-up eggs instead of scrambled. Serve the eggs on top of the steak and let the yolks run over for added richness.

PER SERVING: Calories: 795; Fat: 63g; Carbohydrates: 3g; Protein: 53g; Sodium: 1,662mg; Iron: 6mg

BACON, EGG, AND CHEESE CUPS

SERVES 4 / PREP TIME: 10 minutes / **COOK TIME:** 30 minutes

Having quick, easy recipes that fit your diet needs—but require low effort—are essential. Cook this bacon, egg, and cheese cup recipe for a single sitting or double the batch for weekly breakfast meal prep.

8 bacon slices

3 tablespoons
  salted butter

10 eggs

2 teaspoons sea salt

1 teaspoon freshly ground
  black pepper

½ cup shredded
  cheddar cheese

1 Preheat the oven to 375°F. Line a baking sheet with parchment paper and place the bacon on it. Cook for 15 minutes, flipping at the halfway point.

2 Meanwhile, grease a 12-cup muffin tin thoroughly with the butter.

3 In a large bowl, whisk the eggs until beaten. Add the salt, pepper, and cheese. Whisk until combined. Divide the mixture evenly among the cups in the muffin tin.

4 Remove the bacon from the oven. (It should be about three-quarters cooked at this point.) Chop into small pieces and sprinkle evenly atop each egg cup.

5 Bake for 10 to 13 minutes or until browned and set. Cool for 1 to 2 minutes on a wire rack before removing the egg cups from the tin. (You may need to run a knife around the edges to help get them out.)

6 Serve hot or store in an airtight container in the refrigerator for up to 3 days.

TIP: Use different cheeses such as feta or goat cheese to experiment with new flavors.

PER SERVING (3 EGG CUPS): Calories: 420; Fat: 33g; Carbohydrates: 1g; Protein: 27g; Sodium: 1,306mg; Iron: 2mg

SAUSAGE EGG CUPS

SERVES 4 / PREP TIME: 10 minutes / **COOK TIME:** 25 minutes

This is another great recipe to batch bake for breakfast meal prep. For those who are staying active, are working out, and have high protein demands, the sausage here will be an advantage.

3 tablespoons
  salted butter
8 ounces ground pork
  breakfast sausage
12 eggs

1 Preheat the oven to 325°F. Grease a 12-cup muffin tin thoroughly with the butter.

2 Set a medium sauté pan over medium-high heat. Once hot, cook the sausage, stirring to break up the meat, for 3 to 5 minutes or until partially cooked through. Drain any grease from the pan.

3 In a large bowl, whisk the eggs until beaten. Add the sausage and whisk until combined. Divide the mixture evenly among the cups in the muffin tin.

4 Bake for 18 minutes or until browned and set. Cool for 1 to 2 minutes on a wire rack before removing the egg cups from the tin. (You may need to run a knife around the edges to help get them out.)

5 Serve hot or store in an airtight container in the refrigerator for up to 3 days.

TIP: Switch these up by adding different meats such as ham, ground boar, ground beef, or even ground organ meat.

PER SERVING (3 EGG CUPS): Calories: 487; Fat: 41g; Carbohydrates: 1g; Protein: 27g; Sodium: 696mg; Iron: 3mg

SAUSAGE AND GOAT CHEESE FRITTATA ≡

SERVES 3 / PREP TIME: 15 minutes / **COOK TIME:** 40 minutes

Once you get to the stage of carnivore where you are incorporating dairy and eggs, you can really get creative with your meals, especially at breakfast. This sausage and goat cheese frittata will provide a flavor blast in the morning while also packing a punch of bioavailable nutrients.

Butter, for greasing

8 ounces ground pork or ground boar breakfast sausage

5 eggs

½ teaspoon sea salt

¼ teaspoon freshly ground black pepper

¼ cup goat cheese crumbles

1 Preheat the oven to 350°F. Grease a 9-inch pie dish with butter.

2 Set a medium sauté pan over medium-high heat. Once hot, cook the sausage, stirring to break up the meat, for 5 to 7 minutes or until cooked through. Drain any grease from the pan. Set the sausage aside to cool for 5 minutes.

3 In a large mixing bowl, whisk together the eggs, salt, and pepper. Add the sausage and goat cheese and gently mix. Pour the mixture into the greased pie dish.

4 Bake for about 30 minutes or until the top is golden brown and the center is set.

5 Cool for 10 minutes on a wire rack before cutting into slices.

6 Serve warm or store in an airtight container in the refrigerator for up to 3 days.

TIP: If possible, source your goat cheese or other cheeses from the farmers' market for better quality and to support your local economy.

PER SERVING (⅓ RECIPE): Calories: 417; Fat: 35g; Carbohydrates: 1g; Protein: 23g; Sodium: 918mg; Iron: 3mg

CHAFFLE BREAKFAST SANDWICH

SERVES 2 / PREP TIME: 10 minutes / **COOK TIME:** 15 minutes

Thanks to the chaffle craze, there is now a way to re-create waffles using nothing but animal-based products. To avoid overconsuming dairy, recipes like this should not be staples of a carnivore diet but more of a treat. Enjoy chaffles in moderation when you need a little variety.

8 ounces ground pork
   breakfast sausage
2 eggs
1 cup shredded
   mozzarella cheese

1 Preheat a waffle maker.

2 Form the sausage into 4 patties. Set a medium sauté pan over medium-high heat. Once hot, cook the sausage patties for 2 to 3 minutes on each side or until cooked through. Drain any grease from the pan. Set the sausage aside.

3 In a small mixing bowl, whisk together the eggs and cheese until well mixed.

4 Once the waffle maker is hot; pour half of the batter into the waffle maker. Close the lid and cook for 3 to 4 minutes, or until golden brown. Remove and repeat with the second half of the batter.

5 Cut each chaffle in half, then sandwich 2 sausage patties between 2 chaffle halves. Repeat with the remaining sausage patties and chaffle halves.

6 Serve warm or store in an airtight container in the refrigerator for up to 3 days.

TIP: If you do not have a waffle maker, fry the egg batter in a nonstick pan like a pancake instead.

PER SERVING (1 CHAFFLE SANDWICH): Calories: 632; Fat: 53g; Carbohydrates: 2g; Protein: 35g; Sodium: 1,251mg; Iron: 2mg

BACON AND FETA OMELET

SERVES 1 / PREP TIME: 5 minutes / **COOK TIME:** 25 minutes

Omelets have always been my favorite breakfast food. There are so many variations you can make to help mix them up, and they are one of the few foods you can find at a breakfast diner that isn't loaded with carbs. This bacon and feta omelet is another great recipe for infusing some flavor into your carnivore diet to keep things interesting.

4 bacon slices

2 tablespoons
  salted butter

4 eggs, beaten

¼ cup feta cheese,
  crumbled

1 Preheat the oven to 400°F. Line a baking sheet with parchment paper and place the bacon on it. Cook for 15 minutes (or to desired crispiness), flipping at the halfway point. Remove from the oven and crumble. Set aside.

2 In a medium sauté pan, melt the butter over medium heat.

3 Add the eggs and cook undisturbed for 1 to 2 minutes; then use a heatproof silicone spatula to gently lift the cooked eggs from the edges of the pan. Tilt the pan to allow the uncooked eggs to flow around the edges of the pan.

4 Top with the bacon and feta cheese. Cook for 3 to 4 more minutes until the eggs are set. Fold the omelet in half over the fillings.

5 Serve hot or store in an airtight container in the refrigerator for up to 3 days.

TIP: Try using duck eggs for a unique flavor and a boost of magnesium, calcium, iron, and B vitamins.

PER SERVING: Calories: 804; Fat: 66g; Carbohydrates: 4g; Protein: 46g; Sodium: 1,585mg; Iron: 4mg

EGG AND BACON ROLLUP

SERVES 1 / PREP TIME: 5 minutes / **COOK TIME:** 20 minutes

I think we can all agree that bacon for breakfast hardly feels like a diet. Although it should not necessarily be a staple, bacon is a great source of protein and fat to provide you with some fuel before a morning workout or whatever your day throws at you. Bacon is not the most nutrient-dense food, so it is combined with eggs in this recipe by design. Add red pepper flakes to kick it up a notch.

4 bacon slices
1 tablespoon salted butter
2 eggs, beaten

TIP: If you're enjoying this rollup during week 2 of the meal plan, omit the butter and use a non-stick pan.

TIP: To save time in the morning, make the bacon in advance during week-end meal prep.

1 Preheat the oven to 400°F. Line a baking sheet with parchment paper and place the bacon on it. Cook for 15 minutes (or to desired crispiness), flipping at the halfway point. Remove from the oven and set aside.

2 In a medium sauté pan, melt the butter over medium heat.

3 Add the eggs and cook undisturbed for 1 to 2 minutes; then use a heatproof silicone spatula to gently lift the cooked eggs from the edges of the pan. Tilt the pan to allow the uncooked eggs to flow around the edges of the pan. Continue to cook for 2 to 3 more minutes until the egg resembles a pancake or tortilla and is no longer runny.

4 Slide the egg onto a plate and place the bacon strips toward one end. Roll the egg around the bacon to form a large tube shape.

5 Serve warm or store in an airtight container in the refrigerator for up to 3 days.

PER SERVING: Calories: 460; Fat: 37g; Carbohydrates: 2g; Protein: 28g; Sodium: 1,008mg; Iron: 2mg

SAUSAGE EGG IN A BASKET

SERVES 1 / PREP TIME: 5 minutes / **COOK TIME:** 15 minutes

DAIRY-FREE

Starting your day with more protein is a great way to promote satiety, muscle recovery and growth, and better mental performance. While most carnivore dieters fall in love with the bacon and egg breakfast, swapping bacon for sausage is a great way to boost your protein intake and fuel your day. Use this quick egg-in-a-basket recipe to make your breakfast as unique as it is delicious.

4 ounces ground pork
   breakfast sausage
1 egg

1 Set a small sauté pan over medium heat.

2 On a plate, form the sausage into a disk. Make a 3-inch hole in the center. Be sure the sausage is about 1 inch thick all the way around so it will cook evenly.

3 Place the sausage in the hot pan. Cook for about 4 minutes on each side or until browned and cooked through.

4 Increase the heat to medium-high and add the egg to the center of the sausage. Cover the pan with a lid and cook to your desired doneness. If you prefer a runny yolk, cook for about 2 minutes. If you prefer your egg cooked through, cook for 4 to 5 minutes or until it is no longer runny.

5 Serve immediately or refrigerate in an airtight container for up to 3 days.

TIP: Use a nonstick sauté pan to keep the sausage and egg from sticking, or if you are consuming dairy, use 1 teaspoon of butter to grease the pan.

PER SERVING: Calories: 464; Fat: 40g; Carbohydrates: 1g; Protein: 22g; Sodium: 900mg; Iron: 2mg

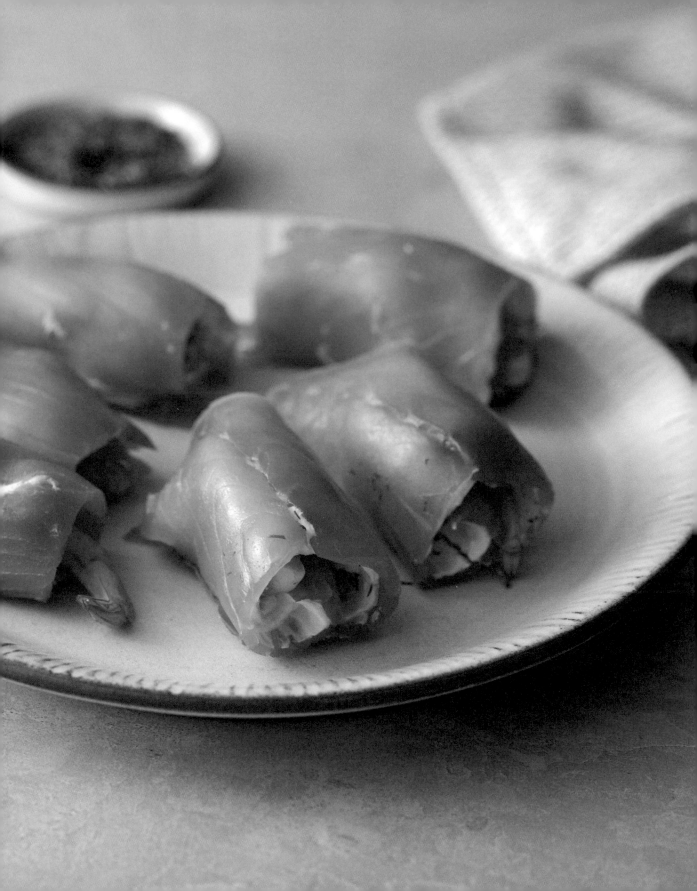

CHAPTER 4

SNACKS, SIDES, AND SALADS

BEEF JERKY

SERVES 5 / PREP TIME: 15 minutes, plus 2 hours to cool / **COOK TIME:** 5 hours

DAIRY-FREE, EGG-FREE

Beef jerky is one of the best carnivore snacks around. The problem is that most packaged beef jerky is loaded with sugar and other preservatives. To get the best-quality beef jerky, make your own at home. If you're a big snacker, keep this on hand to prevent yourself from reaching for junk food.

1 pound (97-percent lean) ground beef

1 teaspoon onion powder

1 teaspoon freshly ground black pepper

1 teaspoon garlic powder

¼ teaspoon curing salt

1 Preheat the oven to 200°F. Line a baking sheet with aluminum foil.

2 In a large bowl, mix together the beef, onion powder, pepper, garlic powder, and curing salt until well combined. Transfer the mixture to a large zip-top plastic bag and cut a ¼-inch hole in one corner.

3 Onto the prepared baking sheet, pipe the meat mixture into 4-inch strips, making rows until you use all of the meat.

4 Bake for 3 to 5 hours, or until the jerky bends but doesn't break. (Check the jerky after 3 hours. If it breaks, it's not done cooking yet.)

5 Cool for 2 hours before storing in an airtight container for up to 1 week.

TIP: Curing salt is used to extend the shelf life of food and prevent or slow the growth of bacteria. You can find it on Amazon or in the spice section of some grocery stores.

PER SERVING (4 STRIPS): Calories: 123; Fat: 5g; Carbohydrates: 1g; Protein: 20g; Sodium: 123mg; Iron: 2mg

CHAFFLE

SERVES 2 / PREP TIME: 5 minutes / **COOK TIME:** 10 minutes

Chaffles have become a really popular low-carb snack over the past few years, but the truth is, many low-carb dieters are overusing this recipe and consuming too much processed dairy. Avoid this by opting for dairy from your local farmers' market and saving this recipe for an occasional treat.

2 eggs

1 cup shredded
  cheddar cheese

1 Preheat a waffle maker.

2 In a small mixing bowl, combine the eggs and cheese. Stir until well mixed.

3 Once the waffle maker is hot, pour half of the batter into the waffle maker. Close the lid and cook for 3 to 4 minutes, or until golden brown. Remove and transfer to a plate. Repeat with the remaining batter.

4 Serve immediately or store in an airtight container in the refrigerator for up to 3 days.

TIP: If you do not have a waffle maker, you can fry the batter in a nonstick pan as you would a pancake.

PER SERVING (1 CHAFFLE): Calories: 301; Fat: 24g; Carbohydrates: 1g; Protein: 20g; Sodium: 435mg; Iron: 1mg

BACON-WRAPPED MOZZARELLA

SERVES 1 / PREP TIME: 1 hour 5 minutes / **COOK TIME:** 15 minutes

EGG-FREE

Even though it involves a long chill time, this recipe makes for a great appetizer option when you have guests visiting and want to keep it carnivore—just increase the ingredient amounts accordingly. When it comes to mozzarella cheese sticks, there is a lot of junk at the grocery store. Seek out mozzarella that has as few ingredients as possible. Although it will still be pasteurized and thus lower in nutrients, you will be avoiding potentially harmful preservatives.

3 mozzarella cheese sticks, halved crosswise

6 bacon slices

1 Line a baking sheet with parchment paper.

2 Wrap each mozzarella stick half with 1 slice of bacon so that the cheese is completely covered. Place them, seam-side down, on the baking sheet and freeze for 1 hour. During the last 10 minutes of chilling, preheat the oven to 400°F.

3 Bake the mozzarella sticks for 15 minutes or until the bacon is crispy and browned.

4 Serve warm or store in an airtight container in the refrigerator for up to 3 days. Enjoy leftovers cold or warmed up in the microwave.

TIP: To spice up the flavor, try using pepper jack cheese.

PER SERVING: Calories: 578; Fat: 43g; Carbohydrates: 3g; Protein: 42g; Sodium: 1,696mg; Iron: 1mg

EGG SALAD

SERVES 1 / PREP TIME: 20 minutes / **COOK TIME:** 15 minutes

My mom used to make egg salad for me all the time growing up, so it holds a special place in my heart. Making your own egg salad using just animal-based fats is a great way to get the benefits of the eggs without the harmful vegetable oils that can drive up inflammation.

3 eggs

2 tablespoons sour cream

1 tablespoon cream cheese, softened

1 teaspoon sea salt

½ teaspoon freshly ground black pepper

1 teaspoon onion powder

1 Carefully place the eggs in a medium saucepan and fill it with enough cold water to cover the eggs by 1 inch. Set the pan over high heat and bring to a boil. Cover with a lid, turn off the heat, and let stand for 12 minutes; then use a slotted spoon to transfer the eggs to a bowl of ice water to cool for 10 minutes.

2 Peel and chop the eggs.

3 In a medium bowl, combine the eggs, sour cream, cream cheese, salt, pepper, and onion powder and mix well.

4 Serve immediately or store in an airtight container in the refrigerator for up to 3 days.

TIP: Add bacon for more fat and flavor.

PER SERVING: Calories: 293; Fat: 22g; Carbohydrates: 4g; Protein: 18g; Sodium: 1,416mg; Iron: 3mg

FRIED DEVILED EGGS

SERVES 2 / PREP TIME: 20 minutes / **COOK TIME:** 20 minutes

This is one of my favorite recipes and something my grandma makes for me all the time. Eggs are a power food due to their protein content and nutrient density. This complete protein source will provide your body with the materials it needs for optimal physical and mental performance. Deviled eggs are also high in fat to help you meet your calorie load and keep you feeling full between meals.

3 eggs

1 tablespoon sour cream

1 teaspoon sea salt

2 tablespoons shredded
   cheddar cheese

1 Carefully place the eggs in a medium saucepan and fill it with enough cold water to cover the eggs by 1 inch. Set the pan over high heat and bring to a boil. Cover with a lid, turn off the heat, and let stand for 12 minutes; then use a slotted spoon to transfer the eggs to a bowl of ice water to cool for 10 minutes.

2 Peel the eggs and cut each in half lengthwise. Scoop out the yolks and place them in a small bowl. Set aside the intact egg white halves on a plate.

3 To the egg yolks, add the sour cream and salt and mix until smooth. Fill each egg white half with about 1 tablespoon of the yolk mixture.

4 Set a sauté pan over medium-high heat. Once hot, make 3 mounds of cheese in the pan, 1 teaspoon of cheese per mound. Place an egg half, yolk-side down, on top of each cheese mound. Cook for 2 to 3 minutes or until the cheese is crispy. Carefully remove the eggs with a spatula and set aside. Repeat with the remaining 3 egg halves.

5 Serve warm or refrigerate in an airtight container for up to 2 days. Enjoy any leftovers cold.

TIP: Add garlic or bacon to boost the flavor of these tasty deviled eggs.

PER SERVING (1½ EGGS): Calories: 148; Fat: 11g; Carbohydrates: 1g; Protein: 11g; Sodium: 736mg; Iron: 1mg

CHEESY "BREADSTICKS"

SERVES 4 / PREP TIME: 5 minutes / **COOK TIME:** 15 minutes

As with other dairy-based recipes, these "breadsticks" should not be a staple of your carnivore diet. That is because cheese is not as nutrient dense as red meat, which is where most of your calories should come from. However, these recipes are a great outlet for when you have a craving and still want to stay on track with the diet.

1 cup shredded
  mozzarella cheese

1 cup shredded
  Parmesan cheese

1 egg

1 Preheat the oven to 350°F. Line a baking sheet with parchment paper.

2 In a large bowl, mix the mozzarella cheese, Parmesan cheese, and egg until well combined. Transfer the mixture to the baking sheet and flatten it into a disk about ½ inch thick.

3 Bake for 15 minutes or until golden brown. Remove from the oven, transfer to a cutting board, and cut into strips with a pizza cutter.

4 Serve warm or store in an airtight container in the refrigerator for up to 4 days.

> **TIP:** For the last few minutes of baking, try putting the baking sheet under the broiler to create a crispier crust.

PER SERVING: Calories: 207; Fat: 14g; Carbohydrates: 4g; Protein: 15g; Sodium: 644mg; Iron: 0mg

CHICKEN, BACON, AND CHEESE PINWHEELS

SERVES 1 / PREP TIME: 5 minutes / **COOK TIME:** 10 minutes

EGG-FREE

Chicken, bacon, and cheese combine to give you a delicious, protein-packed snack. If you are having a difficult time meeting your body's protein demands, make these pinwheels as part of your meal prep and keep them on hand as a snack throughout the week.

½ cup shredded
   mozzarella cheese
¼ cup diced
   cooked chicken
2 bacon slices, cooked
   and crumbled

1 Place a medium nonstick pan over medium-high heat. Once hot, evenly spread the mozzarella into a 5-inch circle. Let it melt slightly; then sprinkle the chicken and bacon evenly on top.

2 When the bottom of the cheese has browned, about 2 minutes, transfer to a plate and let cool for 1 minute. Roll the cheese into a tube and cut into ½-inch-thick circles.

3 Serve the pinwheels warm or store in an airtight container in the refrigerator for up to 3 days.

TIP: Switch up the flavor by using shredded cheddar or shredded pepper jack cheese.

PER SERVING: Calories: 329; Fat: 22g; Carbohydrates: 2g; Protein: 30g; Sodium: 756mg; Iron: 1mg

SALMON AND SHRIMP ROLLUPS

SERVES 2 / PREP TIME: 10 minutes

———————————————————————————————— **EGG-FREE**

Salmon is packed with omega-3 fats and minerals your body needs to function optimally. These salmon and shrimp rollups are a great way to make sure your snacks are providing nutrients—not just calories.

3 ounces sliced
  smoked salmon
2 ounces cream cheese,
  softened
2 teaspoons dried dill
4 ounces cooked peeled
  shrimp, cold

1 Place a piece of smoked salmon on a cutting board. Gently spread a thin layer of cream cheese on top. Lightly sprinkle with the dill.

2 Place about 3 shrimp in a row on top of the cream cheese. Then gently roll the salmon around the shrimp and cut into 1-inch pieces. Repeat with the remaining ingredients.

3 Serve immediately or store in an airtight container in the refrigerator for up to 2 days.

TIP: If the cream cheese is too thick to spread, try adding a teaspoon of water and mixing to thin it out.

PER SERVING: Calories: 221; Fat: 13g; Carbohydrates: 3g; Protein: 23g; Sodium: 927mg; Iron: 1mg

CREAM CHEESE SAUSAGE BALLS

SERVES 3 / PREP TIME: 10 minutes / **COOK TIME:** 30 minutes

EGG-FREE

I first had cream cheese sausage balls at a Super Bowl party with some of my other carnivore friends and loved them. This recipe provides a ton of flavor to help you mix up your diet. Be sure to check the ingredients on store-bought cream cheese to avoid filler ingredients such as cornstarch and food coloring that may hinder your progress.

1 pound ground
   pork sausage

6 ounces cream cheese,
   softened

6 ounces shredded
   cheddar cheese

1 Preheat the oven to 375°F. Line a baking sheet with parchment paper.

2 In a large bowl, combine the sausage, cream cheese, and cheddar and mix well. Use a spoon or small cookie scoop to divide the mixture evenly into 18 balls and roll them in your palms to smooth. Place the balls on the prepared baking sheet.

3 Bake for 30 minutes, or until golden brown and cooked through.

4 Serve warm or store in an airtight container in the refrigerator for up to 3 days.

TIP: Switch up the flavor by using spicy sausage.

PER SERVING (6 BALLS): Calories: 947; Fat: 86g; Carbohydrates: 4g; Protein: 39g; Sodium: 1,677mg; Iron: 2mg

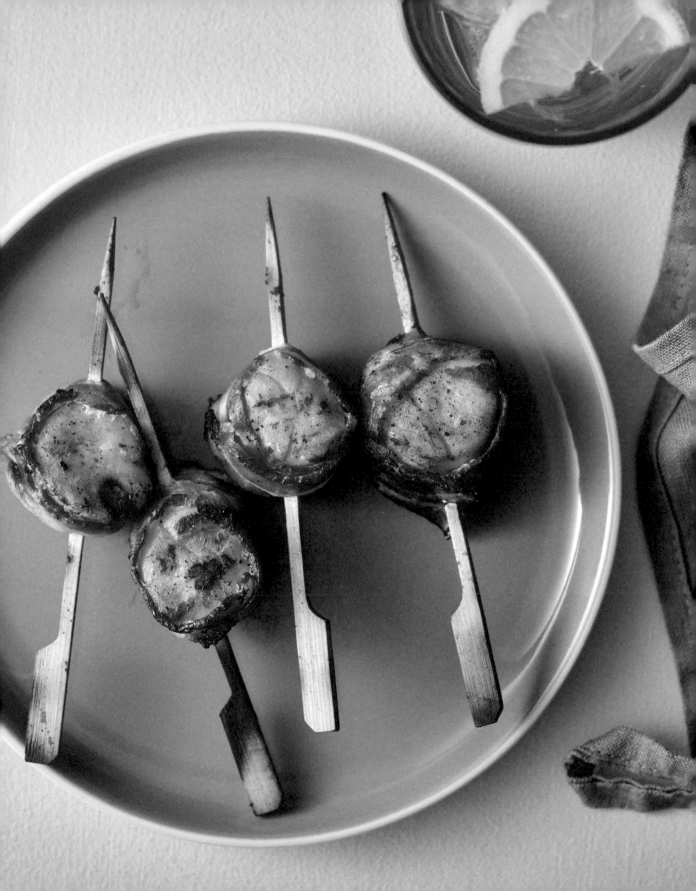

CHAPTER 5

SEAFOOD

SEARED GARLIC SHRIMP

SERVES 1 / PREP TIME: 5 minutes / **COOK TIME:** 5 minutes

———————————————————————————————————— **EGG-FREE**

*Shrimp is a great food to incorporate to diversify your carnivore diet.
In this recipe, you will be searing the shrimp and seasoning with a little
garlic for some additional flavor. Searing the shrimp in butter instead
of deep frying it is a great way to further eliminate inflammatory
omega-6 fats from your diet.*

1 tablespoon salted butter

1 teaspoon garlic powder

1 teaspoon minced
  white onion

4 ounces medium
  peeled and deveined
  shrimp, fresh or frozen
  and thawed

1 In a medium sauté pan, heat the butter, garlic
powder, and minced onion over high heat. Cook
and stir for 1 minute until the butter is melted.

2 Add the shrimp. Cook for 4 minutes or until the
shrimp are pink in color and cooked through.

3 Remove from the heat and serve, or store in
an airtight container in the refrigerator for up
to 3 days.

TIP: Eliminate dairy by grilling the shrimp on a skewer
instead. Chop the onion into 2-inch squares and add them to
the skewer along with the shrimp, season with garlic powder,
and grill for about 2 minutes per side until the onion is
charred and the shrimp is pink.

PER SERVING: Calories: 194; Fat: 13g; Carbohydrates: 4g;
Protein: 16g; Sodium: 735mg; Iron: 0mg

GRILLED SALMON

SERVES 3 / PREP TIME: 5 minutes / **COOK TIME:** 10 minutes

—— **EGG-FREE**

When you think of a carnivore diet, you likely think of red meat. But don't forget that fish falls into the animal-based category and can provide powerful health benefits. Fatty fish such as salmon is a great source of omega-3 fatty acids, which improve inflammatory levels, cell function, and heart health. Salmon is also rich in protein, B vitamins, and potassium, the latter of which is an important electrolyte to replenish on any low-carb diet.

3 tablespoons salted
butter, melted
½ teaspoon sea salt
¼ teaspoon freshly
ground black pepper
1 teaspoon dried dill
1 (1-pound) salmon fillet,
cut into 3 equal portions

1 Preheat a grill to medium heat, around 350°F.

2 In a small bowl, mix the butter, salt, pepper, and dill. Pour the butter mixture over the salmon and evenly coat.

3 Place the salmon onto the preheated grill, skin-side up. Cover and grill undisturbed for about 3 minutes on the first side. Carefully flip the salmon over and cook for another 2 to 3 minutes or until it reaches an internal temperature of 145°F.

4 Serve immediately or store in an airtight container in the refrigerator for up to 3 days.

TIP: You can also bake the salmon in the oven at 350°F for about 10 minutes, or until the internal temperature reaches 145°F.

PER SERVING: Calories: 319; Fat: 21g; Carbohydrates: 0g; Protein: 30g; Sodium: 352mg; Iron: 1mg

BAKED COD

SERVES 1 / PREP TIME: 5 minutes / **COOK TIME:** 15 minutes

EGG-FREE

Growing up, one of my favorite fish to eat was cod. It's much leaner than salmon but is still packed with protein, making this a great meal to change your macros in favor of more protein. Cod, like many other fish, is loaded with choline, a nutrient that plays a major role in optimizing brain function.

1 (4-ounce) cod fillet, thawed if frozen

1 tablespoon salted butter, melted

1 Preheat the oven to 350°F. Line a baking sheet with aluminum foil.

2 Place the cod on the baking sheet and drizzle with the melted butter. Bake for 15 minutes, or until the internal temperature reaches 145°F.

3 Serve immediately or store in an airtight container in the refrigerator for up to 2 days.

TIP: Add spices such as garlic or dill to enhance the flavor.

PER SERVING: Calories: 180; Fat: 12g; Carbohydrates: 0g; Protein: 17g; Sodium: 435mg; Iron: 0mg

BACON SCALLOP SKEWERS

SERVES 1 / PREP TIME: 10 minutes / **COOK TIME:** 15 minutes

DAIRY-FREE, EGG-FREE

Everything is better wrapped in bacon! Scallops are rich in omega-3 fatty acids and magnesium, an electrolyte that is commonly deficient in low-carb diets. Scallops have a very satisfying texture and flavor that are further enhanced by the fat from the bacon.

4 bacon slices

4 scallops

1 Preheat a grill to medium heat, around 350°F.

2 On a disposable aluminum foil pan, arrange the bacon slices in a single layer. Grill the bacon for 3 to 5 minutes or until it is halfway cooked. Remove the foil pan from the grill and allow to cool slightly.

3 Wrap 1 piece of bacon around each scallop and thread onto wooden skewers.

4 Grill the skewers for 6 to 8 minutes or until the scallops are opaque and the bacon is crispy, turning occasionally.

5 Serve immediately or store in an airtight container in the refrigerator for up to 2 days.

TIP: You can also make this recipe on the stovetop. Use a large sauté pan and follow the same instructions, cooking over medium-high heat.

PER SERVING: Calories: 257; Fat: 16g; Carbohydrates: 3g; Protein: 23g; Sodium: 1,010mg; Iron: 1mg

BROWN BUTTER MAHI-MAHI

SERVES 1 / PREP TIME: 10 minutes / **COOK TIME:** 15 minutes

EGG-FREE

I took my first deep-sea fishing trip last year and got to enjoy catching and eating fresh-caught mahi-mahi. This fish is loaded with protein at almost 32 grams per 6 ounces. Mahi-mahi is much leaner than other fish, which is why this recipe adds a little fat in the form of butter.

1 (6-ounce)
  mahi-mahi fillet
5 tablespoons salted
  butter, divided

1 Pat the mahi-mahi fillet dry with a paper towel.

2 In a small sauté pan, melt 1 tablespoon of butter over medium-high heat. Add the mahi-mahi and sear for about 3 minutes per side. Transfer the fish to a plate.

3 To the skillet, add the remaining 4 tablespoons of butter. Cook and stir the butter until it has browned, about 8 minutes. Add the mahi-mahi back to the pan and coat in the browned butter until warm and covered.

4 Serve immediately or store in an airtight container in the refrigerator for up to 2 days.

TIP: Add garlic and dill to boost the flavor.

PER SERVING: Calories: 664; Fat: 60g; Carbohydrates: 0g; Protein: 32g; Sodium: 572mg; Iron: 0mg

BLACKENED SHRIMP

SERVES 2 / PREP TIME: 5 minutes / **COOK TIME:** 10 minutes

EGG-FREE

Shrimp is rich in omega-3 fatty acids and the antioxidant astaxanthin. Catching shrimp can be pretty destructive to the environment, so when it comes to sourcing it, opt for domestic wild-caught or domestically farmed shrimp to support more sustainable practices and protect our ocean floors.

1 pound shrimp, peeled and deveined

1 tablespoon paprika

2 teaspoons garlic powder

2 teaspoons onion powder

½ teaspoon dried oregano

½ teaspoon dried basil

1 teaspoon dried thyme

1 teaspoon sea salt

¼ teaspoon freshly ground black pepper

¼ teaspoon cayenne pepper

2 tablespoons salted butter, melted

1 Pat the shrimp dry with a paper towel and place them in a medium mixing bowl.

2 In a small bowl, mix together the paprika, garlic powder, onion powder, oregano, basil, thyme, salt, black pepper, and cayenne pepper until well blended.

3 Add the melted butter to the shrimp and toss to coat. Sprinkle the seasoning over the shrimp and gently mix until evenly covered.

4 Set a large sauté pan over medium-high heat. Once hot, place the shrimp in the pan in one layer. Cook for about 3 minutes until the shrimp are pink and opaque. Flip to the other side and continue cooking for another 3 minutes until the shrimp are cooked through.

5 Serve immediately or store in an airtight container in the refrigerator for up to 2 days.

TIP: Use the grill instead and thread the shrimp on metal skewers. Grill at 350°F for 2 minutes per side until pink and charred.

PER SERVING: Calories: 325; Fat: 13g; Carbohydrates: 7g; Protein: 47g; Sodium: 949mg; Iron: 3mg

GARLIC-AND-HERB-ROASTED SARDINES

SERVES 4 / PREP TIME: 15 minutes / **COOK TIME:** 20 minutes

EGG-FREE

Sardines have been a staple in my diet for a long time due to their nutrient density. Loaded with omega-3 fatty acids, vitamin D, B vitamins, and calcium, sardines are a great seafood option due to their low toxin and heavy metal concentrations.

1 pound fresh sardines

2 teaspoons garlic powder

1 tablespoon
  dried oregano

1 tablespoon dried parsley

½ teaspoon freshly
  ground black pepper

5 tablespoons salted
  butter, melted

1 Preheat the oven to 425°F. Line a baking sheet with aluminum foil.

2 Clean the sardines and rinse them well; then pat them dry.

3 In a large bowl, combine the garlic powder, oregano, parsley, pepper, and butter. Add the sardines to the bowl and mix gently until all of the sardines are coated.

4 Place the sardines on the prepared baking sheet in a single layer. Drizzle any leftover seasoning over the fish.

5 Roast for 17 minutes or until the sardines begin to crisp and brown.

6 Transfer the roasted sardines to a plate and serve warm or store in an airtight container in the refrigerator for up to 2 days.

TIP: If you don't have access to fresh sardines, opt for canned sardines in water. Avoid sardines in olive or canola oil.

PER SERVING: Calories: 356; Fat: 30g; Carbohydrates: 2g; Protein: 19g; Sodium: 200mg; Iron: 2mg

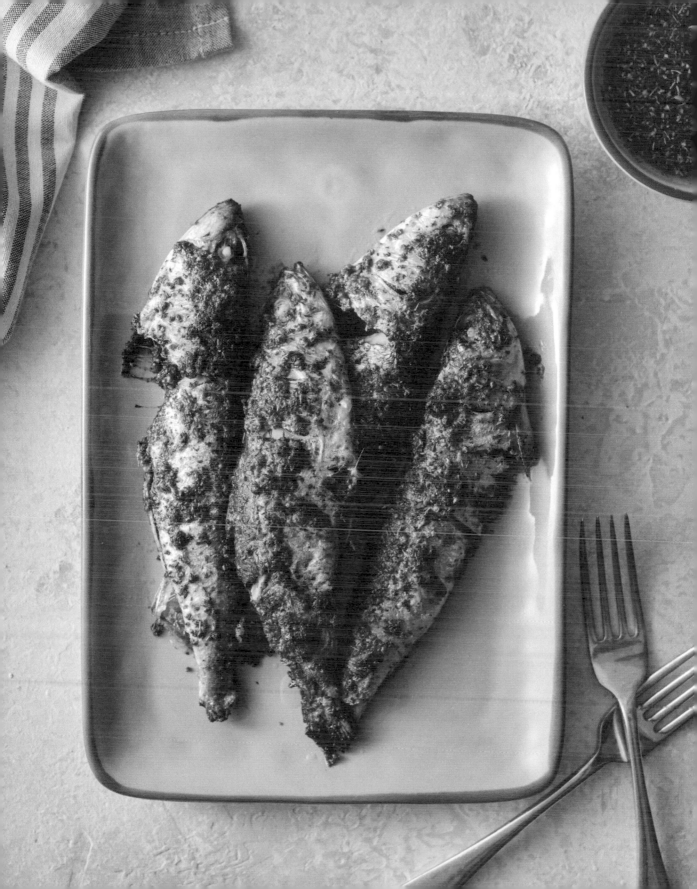

TUNA CHAFFLE MELT

SERVES 2 / PREP TIME: 5 minutes / **COOK TIME:** 15 minutes

Craving a tuna melt? Use this chaffle recipe to create an animal-based version. Tuna is high in protein but low in fat, so this recipe adds eggs and cheese to up the healthy fat content. When sourcing tuna, look for pole-caught, which tends to be smaller and is less likely to be contaminated with heavy metals.

2 eggs

1 cup shredded
  cheddar cheese

5 ounces canned
  tuna, drained

2 slices mozzarella

1 Preheat a waffle maker.

2 In a small mixing bowl, combine the eggs and cheddar cheese until well mixed. Pour half of the batter into the waffle maker. Cook for 3 to 4 minutes or until golden brown. Remove and repeat with the remaining batter.

3 Cut each chaffle in half and divide the tuna evenly between 2 of the chaffle halves. Top each portion of tuna with a slice of mozzarella cheese and the other half of the chaffle. Return to the waffle maker and heat through, about 1 to 2 minutes.

4 Serve warm or store in an airtight container in the refrigerator for up to 2 days.

TIP: If you do not have a waffle maker, fry the chaffle batter in a nonstick pan as you would a pancake.

PER SERVING: Calories: 447; Fat: 31g; Carbohydrates: 2g; Protein: 40g; Sodium: 788mg; Iron: 2mg

BACON-WRAPPED SHRIMP

SERVES 3 / PREP TIME: 10 minutes / **COOK TIME:** 15 minutes

DAIRY-FREE, EGG-FREE

This is one of my favorite appetizers to serve when having guests over for dinner. Whether you are carnivore or not, bacon-wrapped shrimp is a delicious, protein-packed treat. Use this recipe to boost flavor and keep your carnivore diet interesting.

1 pound shrimp, peeled and deveined

8 bacon slices, halved crosswise

1 Preheat the oven to 400°F. Set an oven-safe wire rack over a baking sheet (or line a baking sheet with aluminum foil).

2 Wrap each shrimp with half a slice of bacon and insert a toothpick to secure it. Place the shrimp on the wire rack.

3 Bake for about 15 minutes or until the bacon is crispy and the shrimp is opaque.

4 Serve warm or store in an airtight container in the refrigerator for up to 2 days.

TIP: Try not to overlap the bacon on the shrimp or not all of the bacon will get crispy.

PER SERVING: Calories: 272; Fat: 12g; Carbohydrates: 1g; Protein: 41g; Sodium: 696mg; Iron: 1mg

PARMESAN-CRUSTED COD

SERVES 1 / PREP TIME: 5 minutes / **COOK TIME:** 15 minutes

EGG-FREE

White fish such as cod is much lower in fat than salmon, but it still packs a good protein punch. The lower fat content of cod can make it pretty simple flavor-wise, which is why I recommend sprucing it up with a Parmesan crust in this recipe. This approach will also help improve the texture of the cod by adding a crispy touch.

1 (8-ounce) cod fillet

1 tablespoon salted
    butter, melted

¼ cup shredded
    Parmesan cheese

1 Preheat the oven to 400°F.

2 Place the fish in a small baking dish. Drizzle with the butter and pack the Parmesan on top, pressing to adhere the cheese to the fish.

3 Bake for 12 minutes or until the fish begins to flake.

4 Serve warm or store in an airtight container in the refrigerator for up to 2 days.

TIP: You can also make this on the grill. Combine the butter and cod in a foil packet and place on a 400°F grill. Cook for 6 minutes; then flip the packet and cook for another 4 minutes. Remove from the heat, carefully open the foil packet, and top with the Parmesan. Place back on the grill and cook until the cheese begins to brown, about 4 minutes.

PER SERVING: Calories: 393; Fat: 20g; Carbohydrates: 3g; Protein: 48g; Sodium: 665mg; Iron: 1mg

CREAMY GARLIC SHRIMP

SERVES 3 / PREP TIME: 5 minutes / **COOK TIME:** 10 minutes

EGG-FREE

Not all carnivore dieters need to eliminate everything except meat. Many can reap the benefits of carnivore while still enjoying seasonings and dairy. If you're one of those people, this creamy garlic shrimp recipe is a must-try.

5 tablespoons
  salted butter
1 pound shrimp, peeled
  and deveined
1 teaspoon sea salt
½ teaspoon freshly
  ground black pepper
1 tablespoon
  garlic powder
1 cup heavy
  (whipping) cream
½ cup grated
  Parmesan cheese

1 In a large sauté pan, melt the butter over medium-high heat. Add the shrimp and sprinkle evenly with the salt, pepper, and garlic powder. Cook for 2 to 3 minutes per side until the shrimp is pink and opaque. Remove from the pan and set aside.

2 To the pan, add the cream and Parmesan cheese. Reduce the heat to medium and bring to a simmer until the cheese is melted. Return the shrimp to the pan and coat with the creamy sauce until heated through.

3 Serve warm or store in an airtight container in the refrigerator for up to 2 days.

TIP: Add herbs like parsley to make this dish even more flavorful.

PER SERVING: Calories: 653; Fat: 54g; Carbohydrates: /g; Protein: 37g; Sodium: 1,052mg; Iron: 1mg

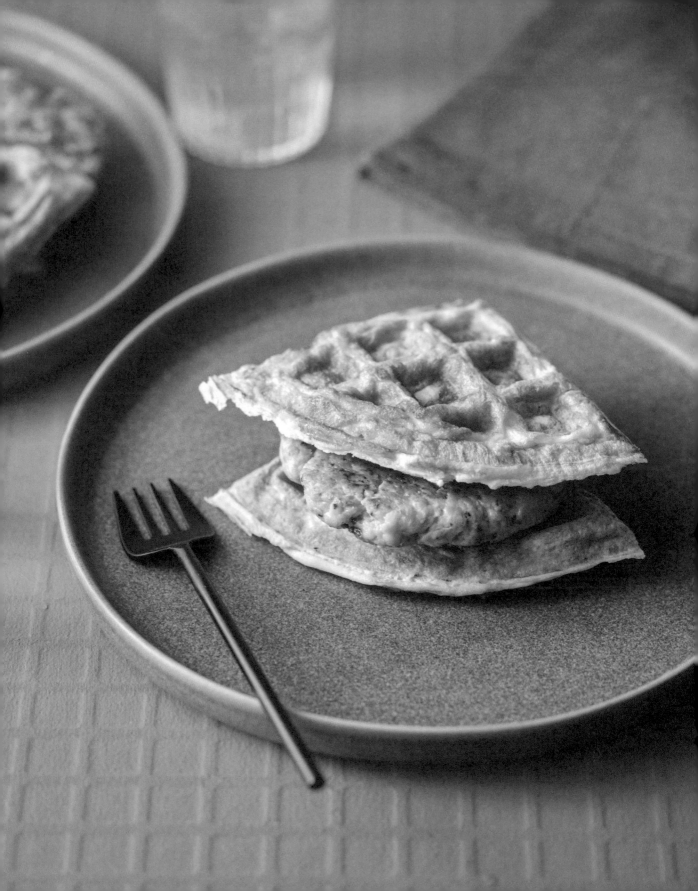

CHAPTER 6
CHICKEN

SPATCHCOCK CHICKEN

SERVES 4 / PREP TIME: 1 hour / **COOK TIME:** 50 minutes

EGG-FREE

I'll be honest: I'm not a huge chicken guy. For years, I followed a low-fat diet that consisted of a lot of chicken with little flavor, so now I would much rather reach for some red meat. But chicken is a great source of protein and helps diversify your carnivore diet. With recipes like this and others in this chapter, you won't have to worry about a lack of flavor.

1 (5-pound) whole chicken

7 tablespoons salted butter, softened

2 tablespoons dried parsley

1 teaspoon Italian seasoning

1 tablespoon garlic powder

2 teaspoons sea salt

1 teaspoon freshly ground black pepper

1. Let the chicken rest for 30 minutes at room temperature. This helps ensure that the chicken cooks evenly.

2. Preheat the oven to 450°F. Line a baking sheet with aluminum foil, and place an oven-safe wire rack over it (or just use a foil-lined baking sheet).

3. Place the chicken on a cutting board, breast-side down. Using kitchen shears or a chef's knife, cut on each side of the spine and remove it. Use your hands to open the chicken like a book; then flip it over. Use the heel of your hand to push down on each chicken breast. This will crush the breastbone and allow the chicken to lie flat. Transfer the chicken to the baking sheet, breast-side up. Tuck the wing tips under so they do not burn.

4. In a small bowl, combine the butter, parsley, Italian seasoning, and garlic powder. Run your hands under the chicken skin on the breast and legs to separate it from the chicken. Rub the butter mixture underneath the skin and spread it around as much as possible. Season the outside of the chicken evenly with the salt and pepper.

5 Place the chicken, breast-side up, onto the rack above the baking sheet and place the whole thing into the oven. Roast for 40 to 50 minutes or until the thickest part of the breast reaches 160°F. Let the chicken rest, uncovered, for 20 minutes after removing it from the oven, during which time it will reach 165°F and retain its juices.

6 Once the chicken has rested, cut as desired and serve.

7 Store leftovers in an airtight container in the refrigerator for up to 3 days.

TIP: To try new flavors, add other spices like chili powder to the butter.

PER SERVING: Calories: 728; Fat: 57g; Carbohydrates: 3g; Protein: 50g; Sodium: 1,003mg; Iron: 2mg

OVER-ROASTED CHICKEN WINGS

SERVES 2 / PREP TIME: 10 minutes / **COOK TIME:** 35 minutes

DAIRY-FREE, EGG-FREE

It's tough to find a chicken wing restaurant that doesn't bread its wings, fry them in vegetable oils, or cover them in sugary sauces. These home-cooked, oven-roasted wings will eliminate all of those issues and leave you with a delicious source of protein to help you meet the macro-nutrient demands of your carnivore diet.

8 whole chicken wings

1 teaspoon garlic powder

1 teaspoon sea salt

½ teaspoon onion powder

1 Preheat the oven to 425°F. Line a baking sheet with aluminum foil.

2 Cut the wings at the joint to separate the tips. Remove and discard the tips.

3 In a medium bowl, combine the garlic powder, salt, and onion powder. Add the chicken wings and toss until evenly coated. Place the wings on the prepared baking sheet.

4 Bake for 35 minutes or until the wings are golden and cooked through.

5 Serve immediately or store in an airtight container in the refrigerator for up to 3 days.

TIP: Add 2 teaspoons of cayenne pepper to give your wings a little kick!

TIP: If buying your wings from a grocery store, look for the kind with the tips already removed and skip step 2. If buying from a farmers' market, you will have to remove them yourself.

PER SERVING: Calories: 827; Fat: 56g; Carbohydrates: 2g; Protein: 75g; Sodium: 943mg; Iron: 2mg

WHOLE BAKED CHICKEN

SERVES 4 / PREP TIME: 1 hour / **COOK TIME:** 1 hour 10 minutes

DAIRY-FREE, EGG-FREE

With chicken, it all comes down to sourcing and preparation. Fried chicken, which is typically low-quality meat breaded and fried in inflammatory vegetable oils, hurts your health. When you buy your chicken locally and bake it, you get high-quality meat that provides a complete source of protein without the harmful toxins.

1 (6-pound) whole chicken
1 tablespoon sea salt

1 Preheat the oven to 400°F. Line a baking sheet with aluminum foil.

2 Place the chicken, breast-side up, on the baking sheet. Tuck the wing tips underneath so they do not burn. Pat the chicken dry with a paper towel and season evenly with the salt. Let rest at room temperature for 30 minutes. This helps ensure that the chicken cooks evenly.

3 Bake for about 1 hour 10 minutes or until the thickest part of the breasts reaches 160°F. Let the chicken rest, covered with foil, for 20 minutes after removing from the oven, during which time it will reach 165°F and retain its juices.

4 Once the chicken has rested, cut as desired and serve.

5 Store leftovers in an airtight container in the refrigerator for up to 3 days.

TIP: Cornish game hens make a good substitute. Follow the same cooking method, but you only need to bake for 45 minutes. The internal temperature will still be 160°F when the bird comes out of the oven.

PER SERVING: Calories: 641; Fat: 44g; Carbohydrates: 0g; Protein: 58g; Sodium: 1,124mg; Iron: 2mg

CHICKEN SALAD CANNOLI

SERVES 2 / PREP TIME: 15 minutes / **COOK TIME:** 20 minutes

EGG-FREE

This is another one of those recipes that can really liven up your carnivore diet. Chicken salad cannoli puts meat, dairy, and seasoning all to use in a meal that is loaded with protein and fat and packed with flavor.

8 bacon slices

1 pound boneless, skinless chicken breasts, cooked and diced

½ cup sour cream

1½ teaspoons sea salt

½ teaspoon freshly ground black pepper

1 teaspoon garlic powder

2 teaspoons dried parsley

1 Preheat the oven to 400°F.

2 Make four 5-inch cylinders out of aluminum foil. Wrap 2 slices of bacon around each cylinder, making sure to overlap the bacon. Place the cylinders, seam-side down, in a baking dish.

3 Bake for about 8 minutes or until one side is crispy; then turn the cylinders and cook the other side until crispy, another 8 minutes. Remove from the oven and place on a paper towel–lined plate to drain and cool.

4 Meanwhile, in a small bowl, combine the chicken, sour cream, salt, pepper, garlic powder, and parsley.

5 Once the bacon is cool, carefully remove the foil cylinders. Use a small spoon to stuff each bacon "cannoli" shell with the chicken salad.

6 Serve immediately or store in an airtight container in the refrigerator for up to 3 days.

TIP: If you have an oven-safe wire rack, set that over a foil-lined baking sheet and use it to cook the bacon instead. This will allow the grease to drain and the bacon to remain crispy. No need to flip the bacon when using this method.

PER SERVING: Calories: 706; Fat: 36g; Carbohydrates: 4g; Protein: 87g; Sodium: 1,843mg; Iron: 3mg

BACON-WRAPPED CHICKEN TENDERS ≡

SERVES 1 / **PREP TIME:** 15 minutes / **COOK TIME:** 30 minutes

_____ **DAIRY-FREE, EGG-FREE**

Traditional chicken tenders are breaded and fried, making them a big "no" on the carnivore diet (or any diet!). But don't worry, you won't miss them when you have this bacon-wrapped chicken tender replacement. (You know you're a carnivore if you replace bread with bacon.)

1 pound chicken tenders
  (about 10 tenders)
10 bacon slices

1 Preheat the oven to 350°F. Line a baking sheet with parchment paper or aluminum foil.

2 Pat the chicken tenders dry with a paper towel. Wrap each tender with 1 slice of bacon and place, seam-side down, on the baking sheet.

3 Bake for about 30 minutes, or until the bacon is crispy and the chicken reaches an internal temperature of 165°F.

4 Serve immediately or store in an airtight container in the refrigerator for up to 3 days.

> **TIP:** Use toothpicks to secure the bacon to the chicken if it's slipping.

PER SERVING: Calories: 1,033; Fat: 48g; Carbohydrates: 2g; Protein: 139g; Sodium: 2,168mg; Iron: 5mg

CHAFFLE CHICKEN BURGER ≡≡≡≡

SERVES 2 / PREP TIME: 15 minutes / **COOK TIME:** 20 minutes

Chaffles to the rescue! Although you shouldn't make them a staple of your diet, chaffles are a great carnivore way to turn up the flavor and switch up the texture of your diet. This chaffle chicken burger is a favorite for game days and house parties and is a great way to increase your lean protein intake.

½ pound ground chicken

1 teaspoon sea salt

½ teaspoon freshly ground black pepper

1 teaspoon garlic powder

2 eggs

1 cup shredded cheddar cheese

1 In a medium bowl, combine the ground chicken, salt, pepper, and garlic powder. Form the mixture into 2 patties and set aside.

2 Set a medium sauté pan over medium heat. Once hot, cook the chicken patties for about 5 minutes on each side until browned and fully cooked, with an internal temperature of 165°F.

3 Meanwhile, preheat a waffle maker.

4 In a small bowl, combine the eggs and cheddar cheese. Pour half of the batter into the waffle maker. Cook for 3 to 4 minutes or until golden brown. Remove and repeat with the remaining batter.

5 Cut each chaffle in half, then sandwich a chicken patty between 2 chaffle halves. Repeat with the remaining chicken patty and chaffle halves.

6 Serve warm or store in an airtight container in the refrigerator for up to 3 days.

TIP: If you do not have a waffle maker, fry the batter in a nonstick pan as you would a pancake.

PER SERVING: Calories: 468; Fat: 33g; Carbohydrates: 2g; Protein: 40g; Sodium: 1,085mg; Iron: 2mg

CHICKEN SKEWERS

SERVES 2 / PREP TIME: 10 minutes / **COOK TIME:** 10 minutes

DAIRY-FREE, EGG-FREE

I would choose grilling outside over cooking in an oven any day of the week. When chicken is on the menu, this is one of my favorite ways to prepare it. The grill provides a crispy texture and smoky taste, and it leaves the chicken so tender that it falls apart.

1 pound boneless, skinless chicken breasts (about 2 breasts)

1 teaspoon sea salt

1 Preheat the grill to 350°F. If not available, place a large sauté pan over medium-high heat.

2 Cut the chicken breasts into 1-inch cubes. Thread an even amount of chicken onto 4 metal skewers and sprinkle evenly with the salt.

3 Place the skewers on the grill (or in the sauté pan) and cook on each side for about 5 minutes or until the internal temperature reaches 165°F.

4 Serve immediately or store in an airtight container in the refrigerator for up to 3 days.

TIP: If using wooden skewers, soak them in water for 30 minutes to prevent them from burning.

PER SERVING: Calories: 247; Fat: 4g; Carbohydrates: 0g; Protein: 50g; Sodium: 697mg; Iron: 2mg

CHEESY CHICKEN QUESADILLA

SERVES 1 / PREP TIME: 5 minutes / **COOK TIME:** 10 minutes

EGG-FREE

Cheese is a great tool to create carnivore versions of the foods you crave. However, most packaged cheeses found at your local grocery store are highly processed, meaning they have fillers and preservatives and lack dairy's beneficial nutrients. Farmers' markets are where you can source the best cheese that comes in its natural form. If you do not have access to a farmers' market, look for packaged dairy options with the fewest number of ingredients possible.

1 cup shredded cheddar cheese, divided

1 (6-ounce) boneless, skinless chicken breast, cooked and diced

1 Set a medium sauté pan over medium-high heat. Once hot, spread ½ cup of cheese into a 5-inch circle in the pan. Cook for about 4 minutes or until crispy. Flip and cook for an additional 2 minutes on the second side. Remove to a plate.

2 Place the remaining ½ cup of cheese in the pan in a 5-inch circle. Once melted, sprinkle the chicken on top. Remove after the bottom gets crispy, about 2 minutes, and add the first cheesy "tortilla" on top.

3 Serve warm or store in an airtight container in the refrigerator for up to 3 days.

TIP: Try different cheeses like pepper jack or mozzarella.

PER SERVING: Calories: 739; Fat: 44g; Carbohydrates: 2g; Protein: 80g; Sodium: 854mg; Iron: 2mg

SLOW COOKER CHICKEN THIGHS

SERVES 4 / PREP TIME: 5 minutes / **COOK TIME:** 3 hours

DAIRY-FREE, EGG-FREE

Slow cooker recipes are invaluable for people with busy schedules. I love using them on Sundays to meal prep for the week. This recipe requires next to no prep time, and I can get a bunch of things done around the house while my food is cooking.

8 chicken thighs

1 cup chicken stock

1 Place the chicken into the slow cooker and pour in the chicken stock.

2 Cover and cook for 3 hours on high or until the internal temperature of the chicken reaches 165°F.

3 Serve warm or store in an airtight container in the refrigerator for up to 3 days.

TIP: Add flavor with fresh herbs such as parsley and thyme.

PER SERVING: Calories: 875; Fat: 65g; Carbohydrates: 3g; Protein: 65g; Sodium: 398mg; Iron: 3mg

CHICKEN MEATBALLS

SERVES 3 / PREP TIME: 10 minutes / **COOK TIME:** 25 minutes

——————————————————————————————————————— **EGG-FREE**

Don't forget that you can personalize your nutrition to help you reach different goals. When I can benefit from increased protein consumption, like when I have been exercising more, I reach for protein-dense meals that I can snag throughout the day whenever I have the appetite for them. These chicken meatballs are one of my go-tos.

1 pound ground chicken

¾ cup grated
  Parmesan cheese

1 teaspoon sea salt

1 teaspoon garlic powder

1 teaspoon onion powder

1 teaspoon paprika

½ teaspoon freshly
  ground black pepper

1 Preheat the oven to 400°F. Line a baking sheet with aluminum foil.

2 In a medium bowl, combine the ground chicken, Parmesan cheese, salt, garlic powder, onion powder, paprika, and pepper and mix well. Form the mixture into 1-inch balls, about 22 in total. Place on the prepared baking pan.

3 Bake for about 25 minutes or until the internal temperature reaches 165°F.

4 Serve warm or store in an airtight container in the refrigerator for up to 3 days.

TIP: Add bits of cooked bacon for more flavor.

PER SERVING: Calories: 330; Fat: 19g; Carbohydrates: 5g; Protein: 34g; Sodium: 931mg; Iron: 2mg

BAKED CHICKEN DRUMSTICKS

SERVES 2 / PREP TIME: 5 minutes / **COOK TIME:** 40 minutes

DAIRY-FREE, EGG-FREE

Another party favorite! Drumsticks are a fattier cut of chicken, which means they provide a lot more flavor. This super-simple recipe only requires a few minutes of prep work. In less than an hour, you'll be enjoying a delicious, protein-rich meal.

1 pound chicken drumsticks

1 teaspoon sea salt

1 Preheat the oven to 400°F. Line a baking sheet with aluminum foil.

2 Place the chicken drumsticks on the baking sheet and pat dry. Sprinkle evenly with the salt and bake for about 40 minutes or until the internal temperature reaches 165°F.

3 Serve or store in an airtight container in the refrigerator for up to 3 days.

TIP: To get a crispier finish, set a large sauté pan over high heat and sear the drumsticks on all sides before baking in the oven.

PER SERVING: Calories: 365; Fat: 21g; Carbohydrates: 0g; Protein: 41g; Sodium: 822mg; Iron: 2mg

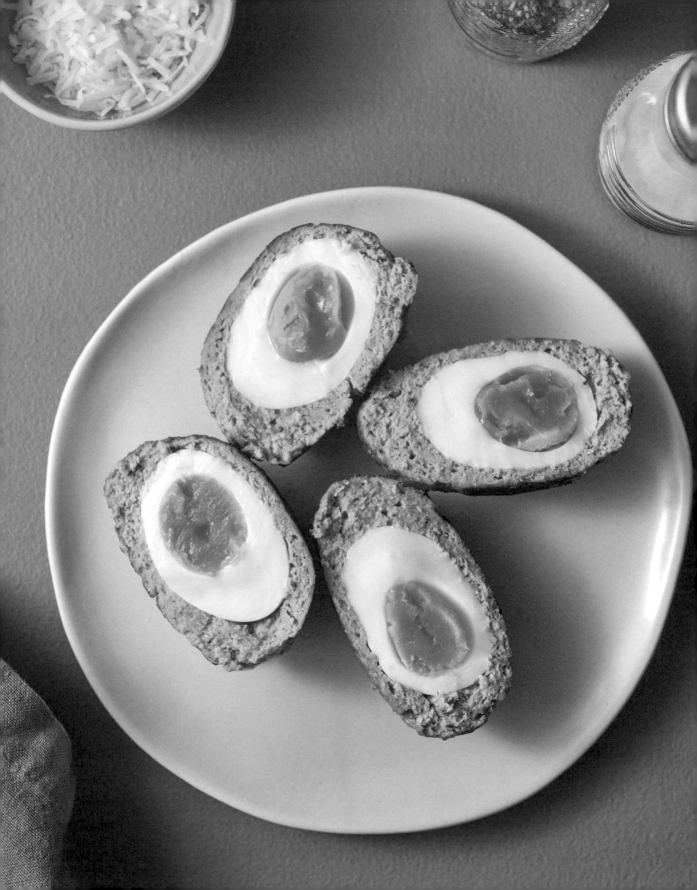

CHAPTER 7

PORK AND BEEF

CHAFFLE PORK BURGER

SERVES 2 / PREP TIME: 15 minutes / **COOK TIME:** 20 minutes

I don't know about you, but I never think of using pork to make a burger. My mind always goes straight to beef. You can eat this patty on its own, but if you are missing the bun and looking for a little change to the all-meat carnivore approach, try this chaffle pork burger.

½ pound ground pork
1 teaspoon sea salt
½ teaspoon freshly
   ground black pepper
1 teaspoon garlic powder
2 eggs
1 cup shredded
   mozzarella cheese

1 In a medium bowl, combine the pork, salt, pepper, and garlic powder. Form the mixture into 2 patties and set aside.

2 Set a medium sauté pan over medium heat. Once hot, cook the patties for about 5 minutes per side until browned and cooked through.

3 Meanwhile, preheat a waffle maker.

4 In a small bowl, combine the eggs and mozzarella cheese. Pour half of the batter into the waffle maker. Cook for 3 to 4 minutes or until golden brown. Remove and repeat with the remaining batter.

5 Cut each chaffle in half, then sandwich a pork patty between two halves. Repeat with the remaining pork patty and chaffle halves.

6 Serve warm or store in an airtight container in the refrigerator for up to 3 days.

TIP: Make this a breakfast sandwich. My favorite toppings are a fried egg and a slice of cheese.

PER SERVING: Calories: 382; Fat: 22g; Carbohydrates: 3g; Protein: 43g; Sodium: 1,080mg; Iron: 2mg

GARLIC BUTTER STEAK BITES

SERVES 1 / PREP TIME: 5 minutes / **COOK TIME:** 10 minutes

——————————————————————————————————————— **EGG-FREE**

This recipe has a special place in my heart because it's from my momma! Buttery steak bites speak for themselves. Delicious, protein-dense, and nutrient-rich steak slathered in some butter will have you forgetting you're even on a diet.

2 tablespoons
salted butter

2 teaspoons garlic powder

1 (8-ounce) rib-eye steak,
cut into ½-inch cubes

1 teaspoon sea salt

½ teaspoon freshly
ground black pepper

1 Set a medium sauté pan over medium-high heat. Once hot, heat the butter and garlic powder and stir until melted and mixed.

2 Season the steak with the salt and pepper; then add to the pan. Sear all sides of the steak cubes and cook to your desired temperature. (About 6 minutes will be well done.)

3 Serve or store in an airtight container in the refrigerator for up to 3 days.

TIP: This recipe is great with any meat, so swap out the steak for your meat of choice.

PER SERVING: Calories: 716; Fat: 58g; Carbohydrates: 5g; Protein: 46g; Sodium: 1,485mg; Iron: 4mg

PULLED PORK

SERVES 3 / PREP TIME: 10 minutes / **COOK TIME:** 4 hours

DAIRY-FREE, EGG-FREE

This is a recipe that is going to take some time, but I promise it will be worth it. If you follow this recipe closely and patiently, the result will be a protein-packed pulled pork dish that is so tender, it will fall apart and melt in your mouth.

4½ teaspoons sea salt

4½ teaspoons paprika

1 teaspoon chili powder

3 teaspoons garlic powder

3 teaspoons
  onion powder

1 pound pork loin

1 Preheat the oven to 225°F.

2 In a small bowl, combine the salt, paprika, chili powder, garlic powder, and onion powder.

3 Place the pork loin in a large roasting pan with the fat layer facing up. Rub the seasoning mix all over the pork. Insert an oven-safe thermometer into the thickest part of the loin.

4 Roast for 3 hours, or until the internal temperature reaches 200°F; then turn the oven off and cook for 1 hour more before removing from the oven.

5 In the roasting pan, use 2 forks to shred the pork.

6 Serve immediately or store in an airtight container in the refrigerator for up to 3 days.

> **TIP:** You can also make this recipe in a slow cooker set on low for 4 hours.

PER SERVING: Calories: 259; Fat: 13g; Carbohydrates: 2g; Protein: 32g; Sodium: 865mg; Iron: 1mg

SLOW COOKER RIBS

SERVES 2 / PREP TIME: 5 minutes / **COOK TIME:** 4 hours

DAIRY-FREE, EGG-FREE

Ribs have been a favorite food of mine since I was a little kid. I remember being treated to them on birthdays and other special occasions. My personal philosophy is that ribs don't require sauce if they are prepared correctly. That's why this recipe calls for dry rub and patience to make sure your finished meat is as flavorful as possible.

1 (3-pound) slab baby
  back ribs

1 teaspoon paprika

1 teaspoon garlic powder

½ teaspoon onion powder

½ teaspoon chili powder

¼ teaspoon ground cumin

1 teaspoon sea salt

¼ cup water

1 Remove the membrane on the back of the ribs and cut them into 4 sections.

2 In a small bowl, mix the paprika, garlic powder, onion powder, chili powder, cumin, and salt. Rub the ribs with the seasoning mix.

3 Pour the water into a slow cooker crock. Add the ribs and cover with the lid. Cook on high for 4 hours or until tender.

4 Serve immediately or store in an airtight container in the refrigerator for up to 3 days.

TIP: To add more texture, after the ribs have finished cooking, heat a large sauté pan over high heat and sear the top of the ribs.

PER SERVING: Calories: 1,500; Fat: 108g; Carbohydrates: 0g; Protein: 126g; Sodium: 570mg; Iron: 2mg

BACON CHEESEBURGER BOMBS ≡≡≡≡

SERVES 3 / **PREP TIME:** 15 minutes / **COOK TIME:** 30 minutes

——————————————————————————————— **EGG-FREE**

Most of my diet consists of red meat because, contrary to popular belief, red meat is one of the most nutrient-dense foods on the planet. It's loaded with protein, fat, B vitamins, and creatine, which help fuel your body during exercise and everyday tasks. These bacon cheeseburger bombs are a fun way to incorporate ground beef into your carnivore diet.

1 pound ground beef

2 teaspoons garlic powder

1 teaspoon onion powder

1 teaspoon sea salt

½ teaspoon freshly ground black pepper

1 (4-ounce) block cheddar cheese, cut into 9 cubes

9 bacon slices

1 Preheat the oven to 375°F. Line a baking sheet with aluminum foil.

2 In a medium bowl, combine the ground beef, garlic powder, onion powder, salt, and pepper and mix until combined. Use a spoon or small cookie scoop to divide the mixture evenly into 9 balls and roll in your palms to smooth.

3 Flatten each ball and place a cube of cheese in the center. Form the meat around the cheese, sealing it and rerolling in your palms.

4 Wrap each ball with a slice of bacon and place it on the foil-lined baking sheet.

5 Bake for 30 minutes or until the beef is cooked through and the bacon is crispy.

6 Serve immediately or store in an airtight container in the refrigerator for up to 3 days.

TIP: Deer and bison also work great in this recipe.

PER SERVING: Calories: 523; Fat: 32g; Carbohydrates: 3g; Protein: 53g; Sodium: 1,314mg; Iron: 4mg

SCOTCH EGGS

SERVES 6 / PREP TIME: 30 minutes / **COOK TIME:** 30 minutes

Traditional Scotch eggs are a novel breakfast item made of boiled eggs wrapped in sausage and bread crumbs and deep fried. This carnivore version is a great way to add a little more flair to your meat and egg breakfast while still staying within the elimination protocol.

6 large eggs

1 pound ground pork breakfast sausage

¼ cup grated Parmesan cheese

1 teaspoon onion powder

1 teaspoon garlic powder

1 teaspoon dried parsley

1 Preheat the oven to 400°F. Line a baking sheet with aluminum foil.

2 Carefully place the eggs in a medium saucepan and fill it with enough cold water to cover the eggs by 1 inch. Set the pan over high heat and bring to a boil. Cover with a lid, turn off the heat, and let stand for 8 minutes; then use a slotted spoon to transfer the eggs to a bowl of ice water to cool for 10 minutes.

3 Peel the eggs and set aside.

4 In a medium bowl, combine the sausage, Parmesan cheese, onion powder, garlic powder, and parsley and mix well. Divide the mixture evenly into 6 balls. Flatten each ball and set an egg in the middle. Wrap the meat around each egg to fully enclose. Place on the prepared baking sheet.

5 Bake for 10 minutes; then flip and bake for another 10 minutes or until the sausage is browned and cooked through.

6 Serve immediately or store in an airtight container in the refrigerator for up to 3 days.

PER SERVING: Calories: 354; Fat: 30g; Carbohydrates: 2g; Protein: 18g; Sodium: 700mg; Iron: 2mg

CHEESEBURGER ON A BACON BUN

SERVES 2 / PREP TIME: 10 minutes / **COOK TIME:** 30 minutes

————————————————————————————————— EGG-FREE

Admittedly, this recipe is a little extravagant. No one really needs a bun made of bacon, but it'll look pretty cool and spark conversation with your friends about this new diet you are following! You could always skip the bells and whistles and just eat a plain ground beef burger, but if you're like me, you'll find this recipe extra satisfying.

12 bacon slices

½ pound ground beef

1 teaspoon garlic powder

1 teaspoon onion powder

1 teaspoon sea salt

½ teaspoon freshly
   ground black pepper

2 slices cheddar cheese

1 Preheat the oven to 400°F. Line a baking sheet with aluminum foil.

2 Cut the slices of bacon in half crosswise. Place 3 half slices next to each other on the baking sheet. Fold the top of the outer 2 slices down about three-quarters of the way; then place another slice of bacon horizontally across the central slice. Flip the folded slices back up; then fold the central slice down halfway. Place another horizontal slice across the outer 2 slices. Flip the central slice back. Finally, fold the outer 2 slices down as far as you can and place 1 more slice of bacon horizontally across the top of the center slice. This process should create a weave pattern, just like you would find on a pie. Repeat this method three more times to create 4 bacon "buns."

3 Place an oven-safe wire rack upside down over the bacon to keep the weaves flat. Bake until the bacon begins to brown, about 20 minutes. Transfer the bacon weaves to a paper towel–lined plate and set aside.

4 In a large bowl, combine the ground beef, garlic powder, onion powder, salt, and pepper. Divide into 2 equal portions and pat into ½-inch-thick patties.

5 Set a medium sauté pan over medium-high heat. Once hot, cook the burgers to your desired doneness (about 4 minutes per side for well done). Just before the burgers finish cooking, place a slice of cheese on top of each patty and cover for 1 minute to melt.

6 Sandwich the cheeseburgers between the bacon "buns" and serve immediately or store in an airtight container in the refrigerator for up to 3 days.

> **TIP:** If you do not have a wire rack, use a smaller baking sheet to keep the bacon from curling up.

PER SERVING: Calories: 594; Fat: 39g; Carbohydrates: 4g; Protein: 55g; Sodium: 1,982mg; Iron: 4mg

CHEESY TACOS

SERVES 2 / PREP TIME: 10 minutes / **COOK TIME:** 25 minutes

— **EGG-FREE**

When Taco Tuesday comes around, remember this recipe. A regular taco is packed with all kinds of processed carbs and oils, but a carnivore taco is all protein, fat, nutrients, and deliciousness.

1 cup shredded
  cheddar cheese
½ pound ground beef
1½ teaspoons
  chili powder
½ teaspoon ground cumin
½ teaspoon sea salt
¼ teaspoon onion powder
¼ teaspoon garlic powder
⅛ teaspoon
  dried oregano
¼ teaspoon paprika
⅛ teaspoon freshly
  ground black pepper
2 tablespoons water

1 Preheat the oven to 350°F. Line a baking sheet with parchment paper.

2 On the prepared baking sheet, place ¼-cup piles of cheese 2 inches apart. Press the cheese down lightly so it makes one layer. Bake for 5 to 7 minutes or until the edges of the cheese are brown. Let cool for 1 to 2 minutes until it is firm but still bendable. Lay the cheese disks over the handle of a spoon that is balanced between two cups to form a taco shape. Let cool completely.

3 Meanwhile, set a medium sauté pan over medium-high heat. Once hot, cook the ground beef until browned, about 10 minutes, stirring to break up the meat. Drain the grease from the pan.

4 Add the chili powder, cumin, salt, onion powder, garlic powder, oregano, paprika, pepper, and water. Stir until combined. Simmer for 5 minutes or until the liquid has cooked off. Add the meat to the taco shells and serve.

5 Store leftovers in an airtight container in the refrigerator for up to 3 days.

PER SERVING: Calories: 389; Fat: 25g; Carbohydrates: 3g; Protein: 38g; Sodium: 790mg; Iron: 4mg

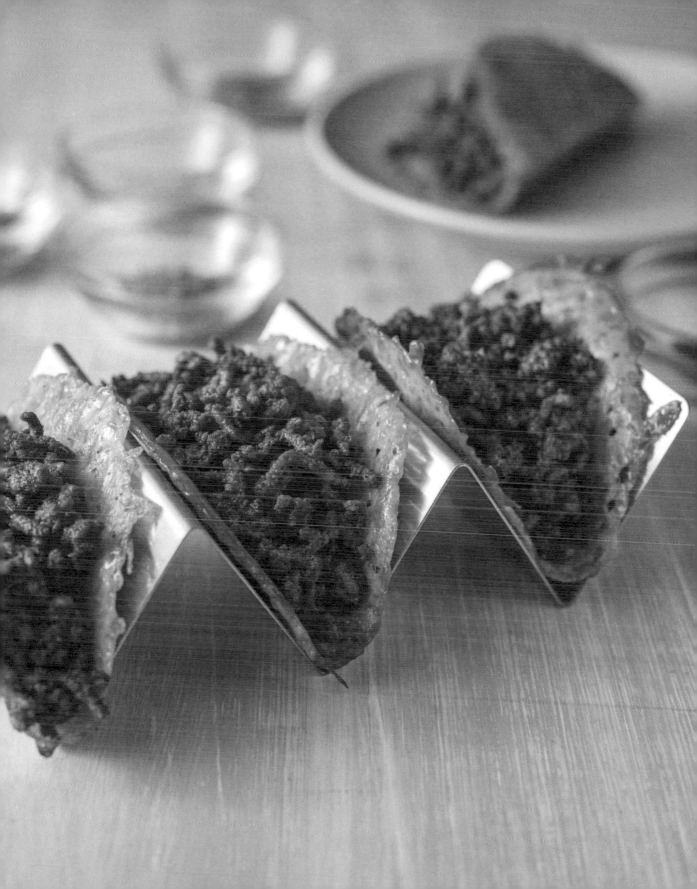

BACON-WRAPPED PORK MEDALLIONS ≡

SERVES 3 / PREP TIME: 10 minutes / **COOK TIME:** 30 minutes

— **DAIRY-FREE, EGG-FREE**

Here's another great appetizer recipe to impress your non-carnivore friends. It's obvious based on the name that this recipe is going to bring the flavor, but it also packs a pretty hefty protein punch with pork tenderloin providing 44 grams per 6 ounces of meat.

1 (1-pound) pork
   tenderloin, cut into 9
   (2-inch) portions
9 bacon slices

1 Preheat the oven to 400°F. Line a baking sheet with aluminum foil.

2 Wrap each pork medallion around the outside edges with a piece of bacon and secure the bacon with a toothpick.

3 Set a large sauté pan over medium-high heat. Once hot, sear each side of the pork medallions for 2 to 3 minutes until golden and transfer to the prepared baking sheet.

4 Bake for 20 minutes or until the pork is cooked through and the bacon is crispy. Remove the toothpicks before serving.

5 Store leftovers in an airtight container in the refrigerator for up to 3 days.

TIP: For extra flavor, add a little garlic butter to the pan when searing.

PER SERVING: Calories: 343; Fat: 17g; Carbohydrates: 0g; Protein: 43g; Sodium: 660mg; Iron: 2mg

SUNNY-SIDE-UP BURGER

SERVES 1 / PREP TIME: 5 minutes / **COOK TIME:** 10 minutes

DAIRY-FREE

Burgers often become a staple on the carnivore diet, but they're made even better by adding a sunny-side-up egg. This burger makes a great meal at breakfast, lunch, or dinner and—with the addition of the egg—can help bump up your protein, fat, and, most importantly, nutrient intake.

5 ounces ground beef

1 egg

1 Set a medium sauté pan over medium-high heat.

2 Form the beef into a patty about 1 inch thick and place into the hot pan. Cook for about 4 minutes until browned; then flip.

3 Crack the egg into the pan alongside the patty. Cover with a lid and cook for 2 minutes until the white is firm; then use a spatula to transfer the egg on top of the burger. Continue to cook, uncovered, for 2 minutes more or until the burger has cooked to your desired doneness. Remove from the pan and serve.

4 If cooking for a future meal, cook the egg over hard and store in an airtight container in the refrigerator for up to 2 days.

TIP: To add variety, experiment with other ground meats such as sausage, bison, or chicken.

PER SERVING: Calories: 257; Fat: 12g; Carbohydrates: 0g; Protein: 37g; Sodium: 165mg; Iron: 4mg

PAN-SEARED BONE-IN RIB EYE ≡≡≡≡≡

SERVES 2 / PREP TIME: 30 minutes / **COOK TIME:** 10 minutes

── **EGG-FREE**

It's no surprise that the rib eye has become the carnivore dieter's holy grail. Not only is it rich in protein, fat, and every micronutrient under the sun, it's one of the best-tasting and textured cuts of steak. Source your red meat from a local farmers' market for better-quality red meat produced under animal agriculture practices that are more ethical and environmentally friendly. (See Resources, page 108, for suggestions for sourcing meat.)

2 bone-in rib-eye steaks
  (about 1 inch thick)
4 tablespoons
  salted butter

1 Remove the rib eyes from the refrigerator for 20 minutes before cooking. Pat the steaks dry with paper towels to remove excess moisture.

2 In a large sauté pan, melt the butter over medium-high heat. Add the rib eyes and cook for about 5 minutes per side, or until they reach an internal temperature of 145°F. Remove and let rest for 5 minutes.

3 Serve immediately or store in an airtight container in the refrigerator for up to 3 days.

TIP: If you're enjoying this steak during week 1 or 2 of the meal plan, omit the butter and use a nonstick pan.

PER SERVING: Calories: 573; Fat: 49g; Carbohydrates: 0g; Protein: 34g; Sodium: 285mg; Iron: 3mg

"BREADED" PORK CHOPS

SERVES 4 / PREP TIME: 10 minutes / **COOK TIME:** 20 minutes

Breaded pork chops are a staple dish in the South, but normally they are wrapped in carby bread crumbs and fried in inflammatory vegetable oil. Make this dish at home to get that same delicious Southern flavor with healthier ingredients.

¼ cup grated
  Parmesan cheese

4 tablespoons pork
  rind crumbs

1 egg

2 teaspoons heavy
  (whipping) cream

4 boneless pork chops

4 tablespoons
  salted butter

1 In a medium bowl, combine the Parmesan cheese and ground pork rinds.

2 In a small bowl, whisk together the egg and heavy cream.

3 Dry the pork chops. Dip a pork chop into the egg mixture and coat both sides. Then dip it in the crumb mixture and set aside on a plate. Repeat with the remaining pork chops.

4 In a large skillet, melt the butter over medium-high heat. Add 2 of the pork chops and cook for about 4 minutes per side or until the internal temperature reaches 145°F. Remove to a paper towel–lined plate. Repeat with the remaining chops.

5 Serve immediately or store in an airtight container in the refrigerator for up to 3 days.

TIP: Drying the pork chops before dipping them in the egg and breading them allows the breading to stick better, which results in a crispier crust.

PER SERVING: Calories: 389; Fat: 22g; Carbohydrates; 1g; Protein: 45g; Sodium: 313mg; Iron: 1mg

CREAMY GARLIC PORK CHOPS

SERVES 3 / PREP TIME: 5 minutes / **COOK TIME:** 15 minutes

EGG-FREE

This delicious, creamy garlic recipe helps infuse additional flavor to pork chops. Like red meat, pork is rich in protein and fat and contains many beneficial nutrients. This recipe is great for summertime grilling and takes no time to prepare and cook.

1 tablespoon salted butter

3 center-cut boneless pork chops (½ inch thick)

½ teaspoon sea salt

¼ teaspoon freshly ground black pepper

3 tablespoons chicken broth

½ cup heavy (whipping) cream

½ ounce cream cheese, softened

¼ cup Parmesan cheese

1½ teaspoons Italian seasoning

1½ teaspoons garlic powder

1 In a large skillet, melt the butter over medium-high heat. Add the pork chops and season with the salt and pepper. Cook each side for about 4 minutes until browned. Remove and set aside.

2 Add the chicken broth to the pan and use a rubber spatula to scrape up all of the browned bits in the pan. Then add the heavy cream, cream cheese, Parmesan cheese, Italian seasoning, and garlic powder, and stir until well combined and the cheeses have melted. Return the pork chops to the pan and bring to a simmer for 5 minutes, until the sauce has thickened.

3 Serve warm or store in an airtight container in the refrigerator for up to 3 days.

> **TIP:** If you like a little heat, try adding some red pepper flakes.

PER SERVING: Calories: 458; Fat: 29g; Carbohydrates: 4g; Protein: 43g; Sodium: 614mg; Iron: 2mg

OVEN-ROASTED BEEF BRISKET

SERVES 5 / **PREP TIME:** 35 minutes / **COOK TIME:** 6 hours

DAIRY-FREE, EGG-FREE

I fell in love with brisket while living in Austin, Texas, for two years. Since moving back to Florida, I have struggled to find anything close to good ole Texas barbecue, so I had to learn to make it myself. This is another great recipe to meal prep. A few minutes of preparation and some slow cooking and you have a few pounds of meat for the week!

2 tablespoons kosher salt

1 teaspoon freshly ground
   black pepper

1½ teaspoons
   garlic powder

1 teaspoon onion powder

1 (3-pound) brisket

1 Preheat the oven to 300°F. Line a baking sheet with aluminum foil.

2 In a small bowl, combine the salt, pepper, garlic powder, and onion powder. Sprinkle all over the brisket and rub it in. Cover the brisket with foil and place in the oven.

3 Roast for about 4 hours or until the thickest part of the brisket reaches 200°F.

4 Uncover the brisket and cook for another 1 to 2 hours. The brisket is done when you can lift it from the middle and the ends bend readily but do not break. You'll know it's done once it holds a temperature close to 200°F for about an hour.

5 Transfer the brisket to a cutting board to rest for 30 minutes. Slice across the grain.

6 Serve immediately or store in an airtight container in the refrigerator for up to 3 days.

TIP: Make a delicious brisket sandwich using Chaffle (page 39) for buns.

PER SERVING: Calories: 364; Fat: 14g; Carbohydrates: 1g; Protein: 59g; Sodium: 1,157mg; Iron: 6mg

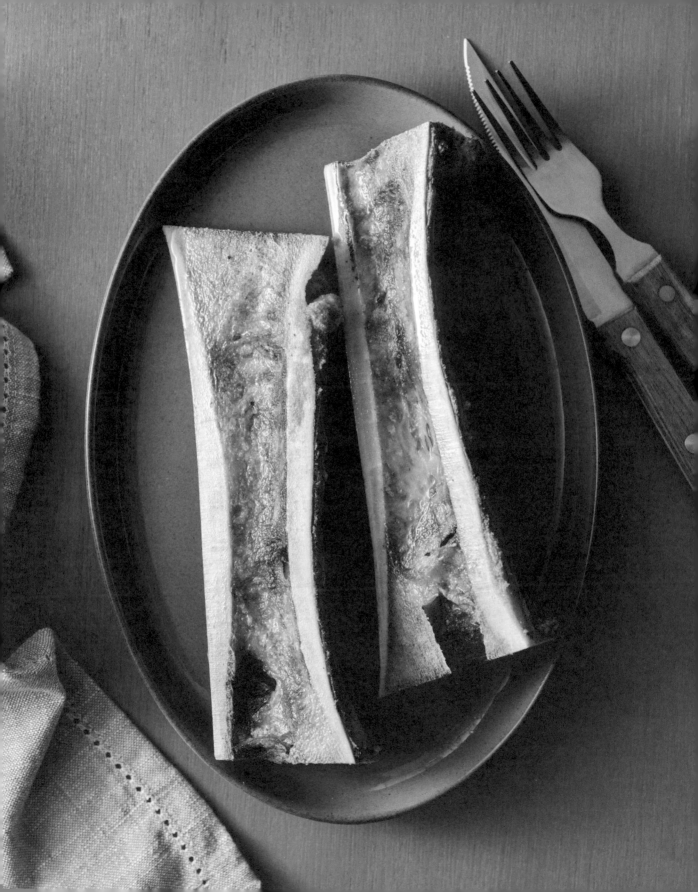

CHAPTER 8

GAME AND OFFAL

BISON JERKY

SERVES 3 / PREP TIME: 10 minutes, plus 2 hours to cool / **COOK TIME:** 5 hours

DAIRY-FREE, EGG-FREE

Beef jerky makes for a great carnivore snack . . . if it's homemade. Most store-bought beef jerky contains added sugar and preservatives. When you make jerky at home, you get all of the protein without the filler. Bison has a very different taste than beef, so this recipe is a nice change of pace.

1 pound ground bison

1 teaspoon onion powder

1 teaspoon freshly ground
   black pepper

1 teaspoon garlic powder

½ teaspoon chili powder
   (optional)

¼ teaspoon curing salt

1 Preheat the oven to 200°F. Line a baking sheet with aluminum foil.

2 In a large bowl, combine the bison, onion powder, black pepper, garlic powder, chili powder (if using), and curing salt, and mix well. Transfer the mixture to a large zip-top plastic bag and cut a ¼-inch hole in one corner.

3 Onto the prepared baking sheet, pipe the meat mixture in 4-inch strips, making rows until you use all of the meat.

4 Bake for 3 to 5 hours, or until the jerky bends but doesn't break. (Check the jerky after 3 hours. If it breaks, it's not done cooking yet.)

5 Cool for 2 hours before storing in an airtight container for up to 1 week.

> **TIP:** If you don't have bison locally, check out Force of Nature Meats online (see Resources, page 108) to support regenerative agriculture.

PER SERVING (6 PIECES): Calories: 227; Fat: 11g;
Carbohydrates: 1g; Protein: 31g; Sodium: 301mg; Iron: 4mg

BACON BUCK BURGERS

SERVES 4 / PREP TIME: 5 minutes / **COOK TIME:** 30 minutes

EGG-FREE

One of the keys to long-term success with carnivore is developing a palate for different types of meat. This will increase the variety of your food selection to help keep things interesting. Venison is a great game meat that is often forgotten about on carnivore. It's a lean protein that's rich in iron and packed with B vitamins. Add some bacon and cheese and you have a brand-new burger flavor in your arsenal.

12 bacon slices
1 pound ground venison
4 slices cheddar cheese

1 Preheat the oven to 400°F. Line a baking sheet with parchment paper and place the bacon on it. Cook for 15 minutes (or to desired crispiness), flipping at the halfway point. Remove from the oven and set aside.

2 Form the venison into 4 patties about ½ inch thick.

3 Set a large sauté pan over medium-high heat. Once hot, cook the burgers for about 7 minutes per side or until thoroughly cooked. Top with a slice of cheese and allow to melt. Place 3 slices of bacon on each patty.

4 Serve immediately or store in an airtight container in the refrigerator for up to 3 days.

TIP: Source your venison locally if you can. Find hunters in your area or take up the craft yourself (with some help and training, of course).

PER SERVING: Calories: 499; Fat: 36g; Carbohydrates: 1g; Protein: 40g; Sodium: 878mg; Iron: 2mg

SAUTÉED BEEF LIVERS

SERVES 3 / **PREP TIME:** 5 minutes / **COOK TIME:** 10 minutes

EGG-FREE

If there's one food I put into the superfoods category, it's organ meat, especially liver, as it's a great source of protein and is loaded with vitamins A, B, and C; iron; potassium; and numerous other key nutrients. It's essentially a carnivore multivitamin. Beef organs are an acquired taste, though, so if you aren't a big fan of eating them with few accompanying flavors, check out some of the other organ meat recipes in this chapter, such as Beef Heart and Liver Meatballs (page 100) or Beef Liver Pâté (page 102).

2 tablespoons
salted butter

1 pound beef livers

1 In a large sauté pan, melt the butter over medium-high heat. Once hot, add the beef livers. Sauté for about 6 minutes, stirring frequently, until browned and firm. Be sure not to overcook; doing so can bring out a pungent taste.

2 Serve immediately or store in an airtight container in the refrigerator for up to 2 days.

TIP: Add some fresh garlic and parsley for extra flavor.

PER SERVING: Calories: 272; Fat: 13g; Carbohydrates: 2g; Protein: 31g; Sodium: 165mg; Iron: 7mg

BEEF HEART SKEWERS

SERVES 2 / **PREP TIME:** 10 minutes / **COOK TIME:** 10 minutes

EGG-FREE

If you think eating beef heart is questionable, you're not alone. I remember the first time I brought one back from the farmers' market; I was pretty intimidated and unsure of how to cook it. Over the years, I have found different ways to prepare it to my liking. Now I keep it in my diet because it's rich in iron, B vitamins, and numerous other nutrients.

1 beef heart, cut into
  1-inch cubes

1 tablespoon salted butter

1 Thread 3 beef heart cubes onto each of the 18 metal skewers.

2 In a large sauté pan, melt the butter over medium-high heat. Add the skewers and cook for about 4 minutes on each side until browned and firm.

3 Serve immediately or store in an airtight container in the refrigerator for up to 2 days.

TIP: If you're enjoying these beef hearts during week 2 of the meal plan, omit the butter and use a nonstick pan. Or cook them on the grill!

PER SERVING (2 SKEWERS): Calories: 559; Fat: 24g; Carbohydrates: 1g; Protein: 80g; Sodium: 490mg; Iron: 20mg

BEEF HEART AND LIVER MEATBALLS ≡

SERVES 4 / PREP TIME: 10 minutes / **COOK TIME:** 25 minutes

── **DAIRY-FREE, EGG-FREE**

Over time, I have acquired a taste for organ meat. My wife . . . not so much. Luckily, we found these incredible ground meat blends that contain a mix of regular meat and organ meat to help us find a happy medium. This is one of the recipes that finally got my wife on board with eating organ meat and made it a lot more enjoyable for me as well.

8 ounces ground beef

4 ounces ground
  beef heart

4 ounces ground liver

1 teaspoon sea salt

1 Preheat the oven to 350°F. Line a baking sheet with aluminum foil.

2 In a medium bowl, mix the ground beef, beef heart, and liver until well combined. Season with the salt. Roll the mixture into 2-inch balls and place them on the prepared baking sheet.

3 Bake for 25 minutes or until the meatballs are firm and cooked through.

4 Serve immediately or store in an airtight container in the refrigerator for up to 3 days.

> **TIP:** You can find blends like this at your local farmers' market or online through Force of Nature Meats (see Resources, page 108).

PER SERVING (6 MEATBALLS): Calories: 140; Fat: 5g; Carbohydrates: 0g; Protein: 22g; Sodium: 376mg; Iron: 5mg

ROASTED BONE MARROW

SERVES 1 / PREP TIME: 5 minutes / **COOK TIME:** 20 minutes

DAIRY-FREE, EGG-FREE

Bone marrow, the carnivore delicacy, has been eaten by humans for thousands of years. Today, it is mostly consumed for its rich buttery taste, but it's also extremely nutrient dense. Bone marrow is loaded with unique nutrients such as glycine and glucosamine, the latter of which promotes joint, hair, skin, nail, and even digestive health.

1 beef marrow bone, halved crosswise

1 Preheat the oven to 450°F. Line a baking sheet with aluminum foil and place the bones onto it, marrow-side up.

2 Roast for 18 minutes or until there is no resistance when a toothpick is inserted into the center of the marrow.

3 Serve immediately with a spoon to scoop out the roasted marrow.

TIP: Bone marrow provides a very small serving, so be sure to add this as a side to any of your carnivore meals.

PER SERVING: Calories: 330; Fat: 36g; Carbohydrates: 0g; Protein: 3g; Sodium: 0mg; Iron: 5mg

BEEF LIVER PÂTÉ

SERVES 4 / **PREP TIME:** 5 minutes, plus 4 hours to chill / **COOK TIME:** 5 minutes

EGG-FREE

The first time I had liver pâté was at the regional farm-to-table restaurant Dai Due in Austin, Texas (highly recommend if you're in the area). This at-home recipe is a close second. Beef liver pâté gives you the perks of beef liver with some added seasoning and cream to improve the taste and texture. Chicken liver is also a great option for this recipe.

6 tablespoons salted butter, divided

½ pound beef liver, sliced thin

1 teaspoon sea salt

½ teaspoon freshly ground black pepper

2 tablespoons heavy (whipping) cream

1 In a large sauté pan, melt 3 tablespoons of butter over high heat. Add the beef liver slices and sear for 1 minute on each side. Remove from the pan and let cool for a few minutes.

2 Transfer the liver slices to a food processor or blender and purée until smooth. While blending, add the remaining 3 tablespoons of butter, the salt, pepper, and heavy cream.

3 Once smooth, remove to an airtight container and refrigerate for at least 4 hours to harden.

4 Store for up to 3 days in the refrigerator.

TIP: If you're enjoying this pâté during week 3 of the meal plan, omit the black pepper.

PER SERVING: Calories: 255; Fat: 22g; Carbohydrates: 2g; Protein: 12g; Sodium: 470mg; Iron: 3mg

SAUTÉED BEEF KIDNEY

SERVES 1 / PREP TIME: 10 minutes / **COOK TIME:** 5 minutes

EGG-FREE

Kidney is another organ meat that packs a powerful nutrient punch—5 grams of protein per ounce plus a ton of B vitamins, vitamin C, iron, zinc, and copper. Beef organs often get a bad reputation for high cholesterol content, but the truth is, you need some cholesterol in your diet, and organ meats such as kidney provide a quality source of it.

2 tablespoons
  salted butter
1 beef kidney, sliced thin

1 In a large sauté pan, melt the butter over medium-high heat. Add the kidney slices. Cook for about 5 minutes, flipping the slices halfway through, until barely any pink remains.

2 Remove from the heat and let rest for 5 minutes. Be careful not to overcook.

3 Serve immediately or store in an airtight container in the refrigerator for up to 2 days.

TIP: If you don't like the taste of kidney, try incorporating it into Beef Heart and Liver Meatballs (page 100) instead.

PER SERVING: Calories: 428; Fat: 30g; Carbohydrates: 1g; Protein: 40g; Sodium: 595mg; Iron: 10mg

BROWN BUTTER CHICKEN HEARTS ≡≡≡

SERVES 4 / PREP TIME: 5 minutes / **COOK TIME:** 5 minutes

——————————————————————————————————————— **EGG-FREE**

Chicken hearts may be one of the better-tasting organ meats on their own. Like beef hearts, chicken hearts are very nutrient dense and provide a great source of protein. All these hearts need is a little butter and a few minutes in a pan and you have a delicious carnivore snack or side.

2 tablespoons
 salted butter

1 pound chicken hearts

1 In a medium sauté pan, melt the butter over high heat and cook until slightly browned. Add the chicken hearts and cook for about 2 minutes, tossing to evenly coat them in butter, until lightly browned. Do not overcook.

2 Serve immediately or store in an airtight container in the refrigerator for up to 2 days.

TIP: For more flavor, try adding seasonings such as fresh or dried garlic or rosemary.

PER SERVING: Calories: 224; Fat: 16g; Carbohydrates: 1g; Protein: 18g; Sodium: 130mg; Iron: 7mg

GARLIC BUTTER FROG LEGS

SERVES 2 / **PREP TIME:** 5 minutes / **COOK TIME:** 10 minutes

EGG-FREE

Your response to this dish tells a lot about where you grew up. I have always been a big fan of frog legs, but they were usually fried. To skip the breading and vegetable oil, try sautéing them in butter and add some seasoning to reap the benefits this protein- and omega-3-fatty-acid-rich carnivore food has to offer.

4 tablespoons
  salted butter

1 tablespoon
  garlic powder

1 tablespoon dried parsley

1 teaspoon sea salt

½ teaspoon freshly
  ground black pepper

8 frog legs

1 Set a large sauté pan over medium-high heat. Once hot, heat the butter, garlic, parsley, salt, and pepper. Cook until the butter has melted and seasonings are combined.

2 Add the frog legs and sauté for about 10 minutes, turning frequently, until they are tender.

3 Serve immediately or store in an airtight container in the refrigerator for up to 2 days.

TIP: You can find frog legs at some local groceries, butchers, seafood providers, and farmers' markets.

PER SERVING: Calories: 352; Fat: 24g; Carbohydrates: 4g; Protein: 31g; Sodium: 872mg; Iron: 3mg

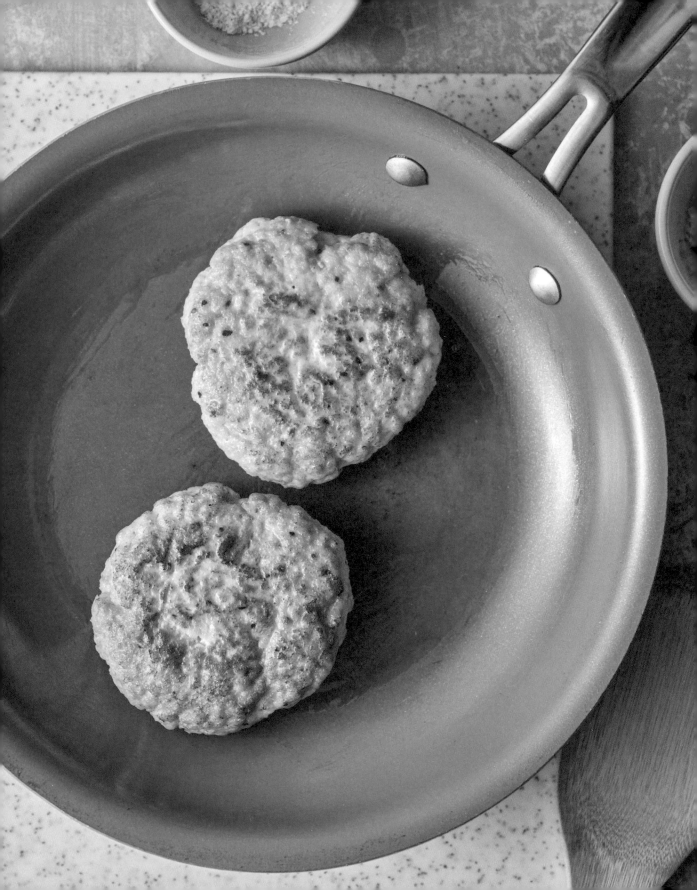

MEASUREMENT CONVERSIONS

VOLUME EQUIVALENTS (LIQUID)

US STANDARD	US STANDARD (OUNCES)	METRIC (APPROX.)
2 tablespoons	1 fl. oz.	30 mL
¼ cup	2 fl. oz.	60 mL
½ cup	4 fl. oz.	120 mL
1 cup	8 fl. oz.	240 mL
1½ cups	12 fl. oz.	355 mL
2 cups or 1 pint	16 fl. oz.	475 mL
4 cups or 1 quart	32 fl. oz.	1 L
1 gallon	128 fl. oz.	4 L

OVEN TEMPERATURES

FAHRENHEIT (F)	CELSIUS (C) (APPROX.)
250°F	120°C
300°F	150°C
325°F	165°C
350°F	180°C
375°F	190°C
400°F	200°C
425°F	220°C
450°F	230°C

VOLUME EQUIVALENTS (DRY)

US STANDARD	METRIC (APPROX.)
⅛ teaspoon	0.5 mL
¼ teaspoon	1 mL
½ teaspoon	2 mL
¾ teaspoon	4 mL
1 teaspoon	5 mL
1 tablespoon	15 mL
¼ cup	59 mL
⅓ cup	79 mL
½ cup	118 mL
⅔ cup	156 mL
¾ cup	177 mL
1 cup	235 mL
2 cups or 1 pint	475 mL
3 cups	700 mL
4 cups or 1 quart	1 L

WEIGHT EQUIVALENTS

US STANDARD	METRIC (APPROX.)
½ ounce	15 g
1 ounce	30 g
2 ounces	60 g
4 ounces	115 g
8 ounces	225 g
12 ounces	340 g
16 ounces or 1 pound	455 g

RESOURCES

BOOKS

The Carnivore Code, **Dr. Paul Saladino, 2020**
   Written by the world's leading expert in carnivore dieting, Dr. Paul Saladino, this book provides science and context around this way of eating.

Food Fix, **Dr. Mark Hyman, 2020**
   What you eat impacts not just you but also the community around you. *Food Fix* highlights the many problems with our food system and what can be done to fix it.

Keto Answers, **Dr. Anthony Gustin and Chris Irvin, 2019**
   I wrote this book with Dr. Gustin to answer all of your questions about keto and the state of ketosis, which also occurs on a carnivore diet.

Sacred Cow, **Robb Wolf and Diana Rodgers, 2020**
   This book debunks the many health, environmental, and ethical misconceptions of eating meat.

WEBSITES

CarnivoreAurelius.com
   More science and mindset content around the carnivore diet, with products to further support this way of eating.

CarnivoreMD.com
   Personal website of the world's leading carnivore, Dr. Paul Saladino.

DietDoctor.com

Medically checked low-carb information site.

TheKetologist.com

My personal website, which contains a whole section dedicated to the carnivore diet.

FOOD AND SUPPLEMENT SOURCES

ButcherBox

A monthly meat subscription box that provides high-quality meat at a more affordable price: ButcherBox.com

Force of Nature Meats

For grass-fed and finished meats including wild boar, venison, elk, bison, beef, and more from a company dedicated to regenerative agricultural practices: ForceofNature.com

LMNT

Offering a variety of electrolyte options in convenient, single-serve packets: DrinkLMNT.com

Near Home

To find a farmers' market near you: TheRealStandard.com

Perfect Keto

Although not strictly carnivore, you can find an array of keto options for collagen and electrolyte options here: PerfectKeto.com

White Oak Pastures

Another outlet with regenerative agriculture and humane animal husbandry at its core, White Oak Pastures is a six-generation family farm that has been in business since 1866: WhiteOakPastures.com

INDEX

ACKNOWLEDGMENTS

A special thanks to my sister, Brittany, for providing the culinary expertise to make these recipes possible. I also want to thank my family for supporting my endeavors, my beautiful wife, Sara, for putting up with my demanding work habits, and Perfect Keto for giving me an outlet to share my content.

ABOUT THE AUTHOR

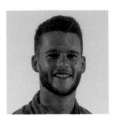 **CHRIS IRVIN, MS,** is a health researcher, writer, and educator focusing on low-carb diets for health and human performance. Chris studied the keto diet for athletic performance and therapeutics in graduate school and has spent the past six years creating low-carb educational content, including the Carnivore Reset program and the Amazon best-selling book *Keto Answers*.Nam dolorpore ipid maximetur maximetur as magniet quas re lictius essum volorest, nes dolorepratur as exeria velecte mollitasi quidelitatem is et et omnis alibus et eumquae commod utem qui aditias dolupti aut quas etur arum eicatat res et optatem ulpa dolores simpore dolest voloria que nis nemperum fugitium at veritat.

Ectem in rehendi psandicae sunt am sinis debitatquiae sunti iustiae voluptaspis moluptas porro temporp orepudi omniatia cusandis di di berum quam volecuptae volut et eossimi nvenihi litiore hentem il et es denihit enienit volorio reprae volum evernatus.

Gent aut por re veligent re nis eate et et et pel int occus magnim quid qui inusciis idebisi alis cus voluptios dollend usapereperae simoluptur, il is maximi, omnis aut utata volor at lis nossum repudam, corio. Ibus, officidus que alitas es des molum eost voluptum et occusto tem cus, nem venturi oriaspiendit aut versperit que por re re ne pro cumque et inturep tatquate nihiliquae estia sum accab ilistiu scienim ad que quia is as dolut alitatiis maio totatium fugitias dist, vent fugiam sequatqui con nempelicae voluptatum conseque imaiorem faccus, te pro volligenimin core volorem. Hitatisto beatius acium comnihil ipsant unti quibus aut harchilia as ma dolorerepre, et, quia distiam fuga. Cae vidunt duci delit, quis erferum, eos quae. Et quunda solupta ad eum, vent a velluptatem alibus, ut repe por sitiiste es aut et ullatecere simosam eum as coritis dolut odi